MAHENDR S. KOCHAR and LYNDA M. DANIELS

Hypertension control

for nurses
and
other health
professionals

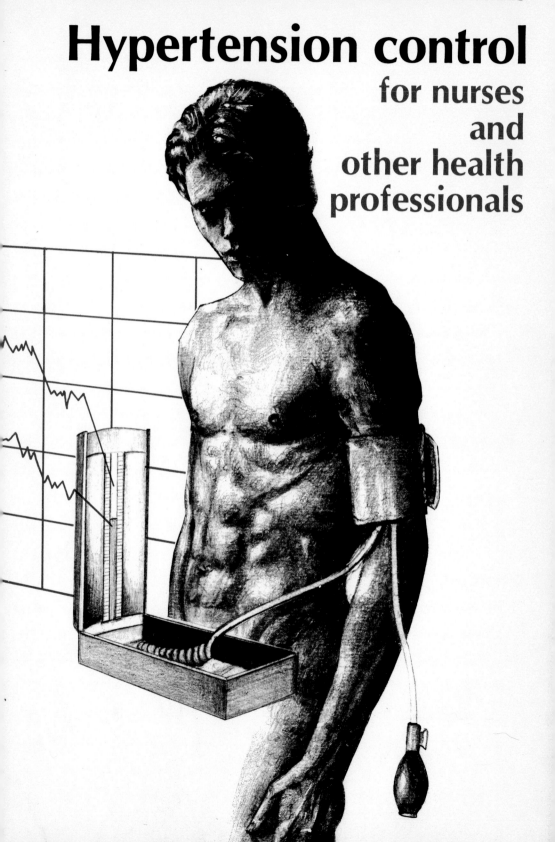

HYPERTENSION CONTROL

for nurses and other health
professionals

HYPERTENSION CONTROL
for nurses and other health professionals

Mahendr S. Kochar
M.D., M.S., M.R.C.P. (London), F.R.C.P. (Canada), F.A.C.P.

Assistant Professor of Medicine and Pharmacology,
The Medical College of Wisconsin;
Director, Milwaukee Blood Pressure Program and
Milwaukee County Medical Complex Hypertension
Clinic at the Downtown Medical and Health Services

Linda M. Daniels, R.N., M.S.N.

Nurse Practitioner and Education Supervisor,
Milwaukee Blood Pressure Program;
Member, Coordinating Committee of the
National High Blood Pressure Education Program

with a foreword by

Harold D. Itskovitz, M.D., F.A.C.P.

Professor of Medicine and Chief, Hypertension Section,
The Medical College of Wisconsin

with 17 illustrations

The C. V. Mosby Company

Saint Louis   1978

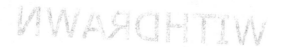

The C. V. Mosby Company
11830 Westline Industrial Drive, St. Louis, Missouri 63141

Library of Congress Cataloging in Publication Data

Kochar, Mahendr S   1943-
   Hypertension control for nurses and other health
professionals.

   Includes bibliographies and index.
   1. Hypertension—Prevention. 2. Hypertension—
Nursing. I. Daniels, Linda M., 1951-   joint author.
II. Title. [DNLM: 1. Hypertension—Prevention and
control—Nursing text. WY152.5 K76h]
RC685.H8K613   616.1′32′0024613   78-3750
ISBN 0-8016-2717-6

GW/M/M 9 8 7 6 5 4 3 2 1

In the memory of my father,
Sardar Sahib Harnam Singh
Mahendr S. Kochar

To my husband—the light,
my family and friends
Linda M. Daniels

FOREWORD

In 1972 the Department of Health, Education, and Welfare launched a national program to help control high blood pressure. This program was instituted in recognition of several obvious public health factors: more than 25% of adult Americans had high blood pressure; hypertension was a prime factor leading to premature death secondary to heart attacks and strokes; appropriate treatment could prevent many of the complications of hypertension and prolong life; most hypertensive Americans were unaware of their problem and untreated.

As the program to control high blood pressure got underway, a number of concepts and problems of process came to the fore that would determine its success: the role of blood pressure screening programs; follow-up procedures; cost-effective evaluation and therapy of hypertension; compliance with therapeutic regimens; professional, patient, and public education. Additionally it was recognized that most individuals with high blood pressure were well and the major concern for these individuals was not treatment of symptoms or sickness but prevention of the arteriosclerotic complications of hypertension. To a large extent preventive measures require acceptance of a healthy life-style and the lifetime use of relatively innocuous drugs for most hypertensive individuals. Heretofore the diagnostic workup and treatment of hypertensive patients were solely the province of physicians. However, from the standpoint of public health, hypertension is primarily a problem of prevention among individuals who are well otherwise. In this context, the care of uncomplicated hypertensive patients is not ideally suited to physicians alone. Physicians are trained to handle acute medical problems and follow up patients with chronic illness who require periodic study and alterations in types and doses of medication. Relative to this training and limited physician time, the care of acute and chronic problems takes precedence over the routine care required by most uncomplicated hypertensive individuals. Thus it becomes appropriate and cost effective for other health professionals to supplement physicians in the care of many hypertensive individuals. A nurse whose knowledge, skills, and disposition can meet this role very well is able to handle most of the medical problems encountered by hypertensive patients and is able to devote more time to their education. As a result hypertensive patients followed up by nurses often manifest better control of blood pressure and adhere better to therapeutic regimens than patients followed up by physicians. This has proved to be the case in numerous published studies. For these reasons, in many physicians' offices and in hospital clinics, nurses are now seeing the bulk of hypertensive patients.

Nursing education has not caught up with these developments. For the most part, school curricula and hospital experiences do not provide sufficient opportunities to the degree that nurses have assumed responsibilities in the care of hypertensive patients. Also nurses' experiences relative to the specific problems of hypertension control—detection, follow-up, education, therapy, complications of hypertension, and their therapy—have been limited, since most hypertensive patients received their care previously by physicians in physicians' offices. This situation has produced the need for a book to help guide nurses in their new role. The present book by Dr. Kochar and Ms. Daniels provides such guidance.

It is unusual for a book concerned with patient care to be coauthored by a physician and a nurse. However, the care of hypertensive individuals now falls on physician-nurse teams, and in this context such coauthorship is ideal. This may presage a trend in health care education whereby many more books concerned with medical problems other than hypertension will also present such combined authorship. Dr. Kochar and Ms. Daniels are uniquely qualified in this area. Dr. Kochar has been trained both as a pharmacologist and a physician specializing in the care of hypertensive patients. He is Project Director of the Milwaukee Program to Control High Blood Pressure, which represents a coordinated community effort to detect and refer hypertensive patients for treatment and to educate the public and professionals about the problems of hypertension. In addition, he has set up and directs a large hypertension treatment clinic for the county of Milwaukee. Ms. Daniels is a nurse practitioner and educator who helped develop the educational component of the Milwaukee Blood Pressure Program. She functions as a consultant to industry, hospitals, and clinics; gives classes; and provides clinical services for patients. She has helped set up a hypertension control clinic that services students and faculty at the University of Wisconsin in Milwaukee.

The authors have presented succinctly the background information that nurses require if they are to treat hypertensive patients. They have covered in logical and understandable fashion the pathogenesis of hypertension, its diagnostic evaluation, and the pharmacology of agents used in its treatment. The book provides many useful insights helpful to the education of hypertensive patients and their families. These can result in better control of the blood pressure, better compliance, and increased patient comfort. In particular a number of excellent outlines and checklists are provided relative to the operation of a hypertension clinic. These checklists can serve as ready reference for most questions and problems that will be encountered by the nurse. The book deserves placement in a prominent location in the hypertension clinic.

The challenges of high blood pressure are great, since so many individuals have this problem, which must be treated for a lifetime. The potential benefits are also great both for increased survival of individual patients and new methods of health care delivery that may arise from the process of hypertension control. Nurses and physicians have important roles working together in meeting these challenges. The present book should prove helpful to both.

Harold D. Itskovitz

PREFACE

The impetus for this manual was in response to a need, the need to control hypertension. The magnitude of the problem of uncontrolled hypertension is enormous. An estimated 35 to 50 million Americans may have hypertension, of which a significant number are undetected and untreated. Also the problem of noncompliance with hypertension therapeutic regimens is extremely pervasive. Complications of hypertension such as heart attack, stroke, and kidney failure rank high blood pressure as the number one health problem in the United States, necessitating increasing demand for comprehensive hypertension education, detection, and control programs.

Physicians, nurses, and other health professionals must address these needs on a priority and collaborative basis. Our purpose is to promote a better scientific understanding of hypertension and provide practical guidelines for its control. Although the major focus is directed to the nurse practitioner, the guidelines presented are applicable to all levels of nursing care functions and settings. Emphasis is placed on control of hypertension through ambulatory, community, private, industrial, and institutional efforts. The allied health care practitioners such as physicians' assistants, pharmacists, optometrists, and paramedics have been assuming increasing roles in hypertension detection and monitoring. This book also offers facts and ideas that will prove useful to these individuals. Physicians in practice may also find the book helpful in regard to counseling of hypertensive patients and facilitating compliance through shared responsibility.

Hypertension Control for Nurses and Other Health Professionals is designed and written with both a medical and nursing perspective. It is based on our experiences with a leading community hypertension control program, an inner-city hypertension clinic, a busy office and consultation practice of hypertension, and an expanding worksite hypertension control program. The term "client" is used for an individual going through various phases of hypertension screening. A person already under medical care is referred to as a "patient."

We recognize that there are a variety of acceptable treatment plans and medications for the control of hypertension. The treatment approach described here has evolved out of our successful experience and incorporates the use of a flexible protocol. This utilizes the talents and resources of the nurse practitioner and paramedical and clerical staff to the fullest extent. The brand names of drugs mentioned are not necessarily better than others. The reader may need to consult sources of up-to-date information for dosages and side effects before prescribing. Certain information vital to the control of hypertension is presented more than once to make it convenient for the reader to understand and remember the subject matter at hand. Much thought was given to the arrangement of contents. The present arrangement seems best suited for smooth readability.

We are profoundly thankful to Dr. Harold D. Itskovitz, Professor of Medicine and Chief of Hypertension Section at the Medical College of Wisconsin, for his encouragement and advice. We also thank Dr. William Hoffman, Director of Student Health Services at the University of Wisconsin at Milwaukee, for sharing with us his experience on worksite management of hypertension. We acknowledge with a deep sense of appreciation the help of the staff of the Milwaukee Blood Pressure Program and the Downtown Medical and Health Services Hypertension Clinic in collecting the information for the book. Last but not least we thank Ms. Mary Striepling and Mrs. Eva Ellis for typing the manuscript.

A special mention of appreciation is given to David L. Daniels, M.D., for the beautiful book cover design and drawing. We also wish to thank Mr. Ted Conte for the illustrations in the book.

Mahendr S. Kochar
Linda M. Daniels

CONTENTS

risk factors, and the contraindications to certain antihypertensive agents; to determine the patient's compliance and adaptation potential; and to develop an understanding of his life-style. The evaluation details pertinent history, appropriate physical examination, and certain laboratory investigations. Special investigations should be undertaken when a particular cause of secondary hypertension is suspected.

5 Treatment of hypertension, 61

Behavioral methods are becoming increasingly popular as adjunctive measures in the treatment of hypertension. The "stepped-care approach" to the treatment of hypertension is proving very useful. Follow-up of a patient in terms of compliance, blood pressure control, and side effects is essential. Treatment of secondary hypertension depends on the cause; in many cases surgical treatment is curative. Management of hypertensive crises often requires intravenous administration of potent antihypertensive drugs.

6 Counseling the hypertensive, 85

Counseling plays a paramount role in the management of a hypertensive patient. All facets of the counseling process and their implications need consideration. The nurse's role and responsibilities are critical. Various teaching strategies may be employed with patients' needs and subsequent compliance as the focus.

7 Compliance with antihypertensive therapy, 110

Patient noncompliance is now being recognized as an extremely pervasive problem in medical and nursing practice. The challenge of this multifactorial problem is enormous. Attempts to define, motivate, manage, and monitor a patient's cooperation with a treatment program are based on several theoretical models.

8 Organization of a clinic for hypertension detection, treatment, and research, 135

The clinic organization and function are aimed at performing high-quality comprehensive hypertension detection and treatment service through various private, institutional, and ambulatory care centers. Utilization of the talents of nurses and paramedical personnel is key to the success of a hypertension clinic. Contributing factors and various approaches to hypertension control are being investigated extensively. Computerized data processing and evaluation methods are easily adaptable.

9 Hypertension control at the work setting, 172

Hypertension screening and treatment at the worksite has proved to be a highly effective and readily adaptable approach to hypertension control. Advantages to both the employer and employee are numerous. The occupational nurse is in a strategic position to detect hypertension and monitor and educate the young working hypertensives. Various models of worksite hypertension control programs provide dramatic opportunity for hypertension control.

CHAPTER 1

Epidemiology and critical issues in hypertension control

Arterial blood pressure is a measurement similar to height and weight. However, the higher the blood pressure the worse the prognosis in terms of morbidity and mortality from its complications. The World Health Organization has defined "hypertension" as blood pressure of 160/95 mm. Hg or above. However, blood pressure levels of 140/90 mm. Hg or above are considered elevated by most experts for individuals under the age of 50 years. For persons older than 50 years of age, blood pressure of 160/95 mm. Hg or higher is considered elevated by most physicians. It has long been known that arterial pressure is influenced by environmental factors, being raised by anger, fear, pain, cold, and exercise.

The variations in pressure found in normal subjects during ordinary, day-to-day living are great. Although the arterial pressure as measured in the physician's office or clinic is generally higher, it is in fact a value that is reasonably replicable, provided that the usual precautions are taken to ensure that the patient is comfortable, resting, quiet and at ease. Blood pressure tends to be lower when recorded by nurses and paramedical personnel than when recorded by a physician. Presumably, patients become apprehensive during physician examination. A more reliable estimate of average blood pressure can be accurately obtained if measured under basal conditions on three separate occasions, with the three readings then averaged.

Labile hypertension is present when an individual manifests periodic elevations in blood pressure. In the absence of sustained hypertension, these patients usually do not develop the serious complications of severe hypertension. However, almost 25% of labile hypertensives proceed to develop sustained hypertension. Patients with labile hypertension should therefore be observed to detect the development of sustained hypertension in its early stages. If other risk factors are present, serious consideration should be given to pharmacologic treatment of labile hypertension in an attempt to keep the blood pressure normal at all times.

PREVALENCE OF HYPERTENSION

Varying figures are available for the prevalence of hypertension. There are definite variations with age, sex, and race.

The National Health Examination Survey of the Public Health Service collected high blood pressure prevalence data in 1962 on a random sample of the United States adult population, ages 18 to 79 years. The study revealed that about 15% of whites and 28% of blacks have a systolic blood pressure greater than or equal to 160 mm. Hg and/or diastolic pressure greater than or equal to 95 mm. Hg. Based on a 1971 Health and Nutrition Examination Survey, it was estimated that there were 24 million hypertensives in the United States. Half of these were unaware of their condition. Of the 12 million who were aware of having elevated blood pressure, only half (6 million) were receiving therapy, but only half this number (3 million) had their blood pressure adequately controlled.

Since 1974 the Milwaukee Blood Pressure Program has screened over 175,000 individuals for hypertension. The criteria for hypertension were as follows: 18 to 49 years old, $\geq 140/90$ mm. Hg; 50 to 59 years old, $\geq 150/95$ mm. Hg; and over the age of 60 years, $\geq 180/100$ mm. Hg. All suspected hypertensives, as indicated

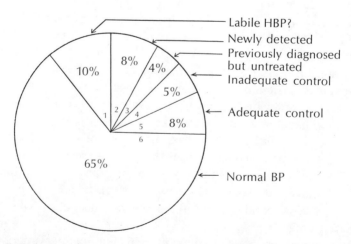

Fig. 1. Prevalence of hypertension in the population screened. N = 106,581.

by two elevated readings, not already on treatment were referred to physicians for evaluation and treatment.

Cumulative data (Fig. 1) revealed that 65% of the population had normal blood pressure. Ten percent were considered to have labile hypertension. These included people who were previously told by their physicians that they had high blood pressure but were found to have normal blood pressure on screening and those with elevated blood pressure readings on one screening but a normal read-

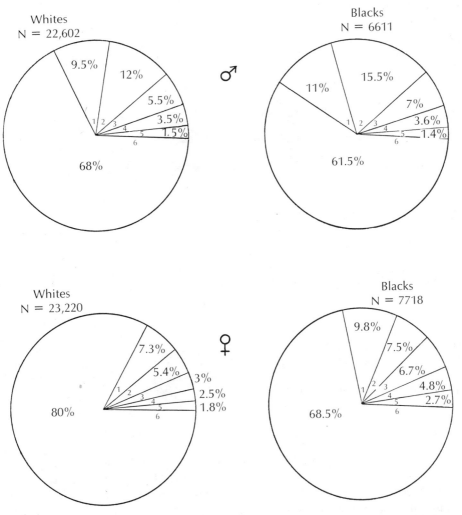

Fig. 2. Prevalence of hypertension in adults 18 to 49 years of age by race and sex. BP ≥ 140/90 mm. Hg. *1,* Labile high blood pressure (?); *2,* newly detected; *3,* previously diagnosed but untreated; *4,* inadequate control; *5,* adequate control; *6,* normal blood pressure.

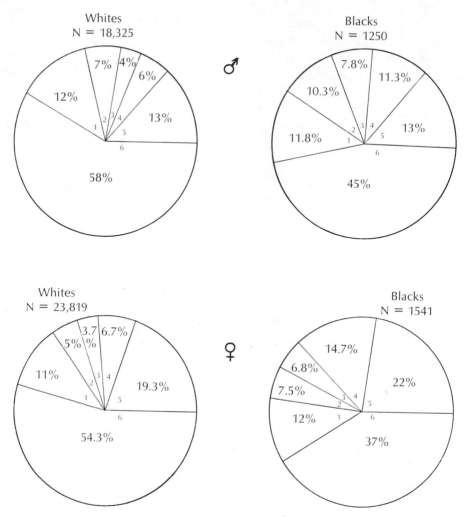

Fig. 3. Prevalence of hypertension in individuals age 50 years and older by race and sex. 50 to 59 years, BP ≥ 150/95 mm. Hg; over 60 years, BP ≥ 180/100 mm. Hg. *1,* Labile high blood pressure (?); *2,* newly detected; *3,* previously diagnosed but untreated; *4,* inadequate control; *5,* adequate control; *6,* normal blood pressure.

ing on two subsequent screenings. Twenty-five percent of the population were found to have persistent hypertension. At the time of screening, half the number of hypertensive patients (13% of the population) said they were receiving treatment. However, 5% of the population had elevated blood pressure despite treatment. Eight percent of the population were found to be hypertensive but had no previous knowledge of the condition. Four percent of the people were aware of hypertension and were confirmed to have elevated blood pressure but were not on treatment.

Among white males under the age of 50 years (Fig. 2), the number of hypertensive patients receiving treatment was considerably lower. More than 17% of the population in this group was found to have untreated hypertension. Among black males under the age of 50 years, more than 22% of the population had untreated hypertension. The prevalence of hypertension in females under the age of 50 years in both black and white categories was not as high, and a larger proportion of these patients were receiving treatment. The prevalence of hypertension increased substantially with age, even though higher levels of blood pressure were used for diagnosing hypertension (Fig. 3). The prevalence of hypertension among blacks over the age of 50 years was more than 50% of the population; however, the majority of hypertensives were being treated.

COMPLICATIONS OF HYPERTENSION

Hypertension is often asymptomatic, especially early in its course. Symptoms usually appear only after complications have occurred. It is therefore necessary to detect hypertension in its earliest stages by measurement of blood pressure and to control it to prevent complications.

The complications of hypertension are devastating. They can be divided into those which are due to hypertension and those which are associated with the accompanying atherosclerosis.

Hypertensive complications

Malignant hypertension is characterized by diastolic blood pressure of 130 mm. Hg or higher, accompanied by retinal hemorrhages, exudates, papilledema, and renal insufficiency. It leads to fibrinoid necrosis of the small arteries and arterioles, which results from the rupture of muscle fibers and enormous exudation of plasma with or without red cells. Stenosis or obliteration of the vessel lumen follows. Later there may be an inflammatory reaction involving all the arterial layers, especially the adventitia. Organs affected are the kidneys, pancreas, adrenal, gut, brain, heart, and liver, generally in that order. The malignant phase may occur in any age group and is related to only the height of arterial pressure, although the rate of rise may also be important. It can be reversed by reducing and controlling the arterial pressure, provided the renal function is intact.

Another complication of elevated blood pressure is *cerebral hemorrhage*, resulting from rupture of miliary aneurysms of the very small cerebral arteries. These aneurysms develop due to elevated blood pressure alone, independent of any atheromatous lesions of the arteries in the brain. They are also known as "Charcot-Bouchard aneurysms" and are caused by rupture of the media and herniation of the intima through this rupture. Thus the wall of the aneurysm consists of only the intima and adventitia. These aneurysms are more common in hypertensives over the age of 40 years. Cerebral hemorrhage as a complication of hypertension is unusually common in Japan for reasons that are not clear.

Congestive heart failure results when the left ventricle reaches its limit of hypertrophy in response to the heavier workload imposed by elevated and rising blood pressure. A fourth heart sound (S_4, atrial, or presystolic gallop) is frequently heard in patients with hypertension. It is produced by presystolic contraction of the atrium pushing blood into the rigid ventricle. The earliest and most useful sign of left ventricular failure is a third heart sound (S_3, ventricular, diastolic, or protodiastolic gallop). It is best heard near the cardiac apex and is caused by vibrations of the dilated and failing ventricle as it begins to fill during diastole. It is heard soon after the second heart sound. At first the heart failure occurs only during exercise, and the patient experiences dyspnea on exertion. Later the ventricle begins to fail at night when the patient is supine, with the consequent increased venous return from the lower extremities. Unless the hypertension is properly treated, the pulmonary capillary pressure rises high enough to produce sufficient pulmonary edema to endanger the patient's life. The most important treatment is to reduce the blood pressure and to maintain that control.

The most devastating but relatively uncommon complication of severe hypertension is the *dissecting aortic aneurysm*. Long-standing, severe hypertension stretches the elastic tissues of the aorta. With prolonged stretching, the elastic fibers may rupture, with subsequent leaking of blood into the aortic wall. During dissection, the patient usually feels intense pain between the shoulder blades. The diagnosis is generally made by a chest x-ray examination, which indicates widening of the aortic shadow, and is confirmed by aortic angiography. The dissection may extend into the major branches of the aorta and lead to rupture of the aorta. It is imperative that blood pressure be controlled within a matter of minutes and monitored closely.

Arteriosclerotic complications

Atherosclerosis is the most common complication of hypertension. It leads to *coronary artery disease,* causing myocardial infarction, and cerebral thrombosis, causing *stroke.* The excessive lateral pressure on the arterial wall probably damages the vascular intima, causing aggregation of platelets forming microthrombi, which later organize. Cholesterol and other lipids are then deposited on these areas, forming plaques. The exact pathogenesis, however, is still disputed. The disease is symptomless until a thrombus closes a vessel to produce ischemia or infarction with death of tissue. Disease of the coronary arteries is the most frequent cause of symptoms, resulting in angina pectoris, myocardial infarction, and sudden death. Disease of the arteries of the neck and circle of Willis results in various forms of stroke. Involvement of the arteries of the leg results in intermittent claudication and gangrene. Narrowing of the renal arteries can make hypertension worse and leads to impaired renal function. The arteries of the upper limbs are more rarely affected. Raised arterial pressure also leads to fatty hyaline thickening of the arterioles, particularly of the kidney. This condition is known as "nephrosclerosis."

The *retinal complications* of hypertension result from the effects of both the elevated blood pressure and arteriosclerosis. They are described in Chapter 3.

√ CARDIOVASCULAR RISK FACTORS

Certain factors predispose to development of atherosclerosis, involving the aorta and large arteries, and arteriosclerosis, involving the smaller arteries, resulting in increased cardiovascular mortality. These risk factors are as follows.

Hypertension. As previously mentioned, hypertension is the major risk factor for development of arteriosclerosis.

Age. The older the subject the more widespread and severe the arteriosclerotic disease. However, in terms of overall life expectancy, a younger person with the same elevation in blood pressure has the more serious condition. For example, a person in whom hypertension develops at 30 years of age has a significantly lesser chance of living to 60 years of age than the person in whom hypertension develops at the age of 55 years.

Sex. Arteriosclerosis is far more common in males than in females. With all other risk factors being equal, females suffer the same degree of severity of arteriosclerosis approximately fifteen years later than males.

Serum cholesterol level. The higher the low-density cholesterol level the greater the risk of coronary heart disease. High concentrations of high-density lipoprotein cholesterol, however, appear to be protective. Other lipid abnormalities such as triglyceride elevation contribute to atherosclerosis; however, their role in atherogenesis is not as well defined as that of cholesterol. About 1 in 4 men and women, ages 45 to 54 years, has an elevated serum cholesterol level of 260 mg or higher. The Framingham study data suggest that in men under 55 years of age, cholesterol levels of 265 mg. and higher are associated with two times the normal coronary disease rate and levels of 300 mg. and higher with three times the normal coronary disease rates.[3]

Race. Not only is hypertension more prevalent in blacks than in whites, but it is also more severe. The vital statistics indicate that the mortality risk in black patients with hypertension is approximately two to six times more than in whites. As a prognostic index, the racial difference applies most importantly to black patients who are less than 50 years old. In blacks, cerebral and renal complications of hypertensive vascular disease are more common than coronary artery disease.

Cigarette smoking. Data show that in hypertensive men 45 to 54 years of age, with elevated serum cholesterol, smoking over 20 cigarettes a day increases coronary death rates three times the normal rate and cerebrovascular death rates seven times the normal. The greater the number of cigarettes smoked in a day the greater the risk of myocardial infarction and stroke. Although cigarette smoking is not etiologically related to hypertension, in terms of mortality from cardiovascular and cerebrovascular diseases, the combination of elevated blood pressure and smoking is considerably more dangerous than elevated blood pressure alone. It is more than additive. Sudden death occurs more frequently in hypertensives who smoke.

Diabetes. Diabetes expedites the process of atherosclerosis and in combination with hypertension may lead to severe cardiovascular and cerebrovascular disease at a relatively early age. Although it remains to be demonstrated that control of hyperglycemia has a significant effect on atherosclerosis, it is prudent to control diabetes as effectively as possible.

Heredity. A history of early death in a parent or sibling from hypertensive complications such as stroke, renal failure, or congestive heart failure indicates that the patient with borderline or mild hypertension will probably progress to a more severe stage. That the familial clustering is due to genetic rather than environmental influence is suggested by observations made on identical twins with hypertension. A close similarity of blood pressure levels is seen in monozygotic twins, whereas in dizygotic twins the blood pressure may differ to the same degree as is found in other siblings.

Obesity. Obesity leads to hypertension and is also believed to be an independent risk factor for the development of atherosclerosis. Whether obesity contributes as a risk factor through hypercholesterolemia or by some other mechanism is not clear.

Alcohol. More than an ounce of alcohol a day can lead to elevated blood pressure. Consumption of excessive amounts of alcohol can also lead to weakening of the heart muscle (cardiomyopathy). Alcohol causes hyperlipidemia and can expedite atherosclerosis. Thus hypertension and excessive alcohol consumption can lead to early and more severe heart disease as compared to hypertension alone.

Sedentary life-style and lack of physical exercise. In a British study, myocardial infarction was found to be more common in bus drivers than bus conductors and in post office clerks than in postmen. The sedentary life-style of bus drivers and postal clerks was believed to increase their chances of having a heart attack. Isometric exercises such as weight lifting and wrestling can lead to elevation in blood pressure, but isotonic and rhythmic exercises help lower the blood pressure by vasodilation.

Emotional stress. It is widely believed that excessive mental strain can lead to hypertension. However, the scientific evidence for this belief is nonconclusive. Sudden emotional shock can lead to excessive production of adrenalin, which can precipitate arrhythmia and cause sudden death in a patient with underlying severe coronary artery disease and electrical instability of the heart. Friedman[2] believes that hard-driven "type A" people are more prone to heart attack than easygoing "type B" individuals.

Hyperuricemia. Elevated uric acid is well correlated with high blood pressure and cardiovascular mortality. As yet there is no evidence that hyperuricemia leads to coronary artery disease. In addition, hypertension does not lead to hyperuricemia or vice versa.

Socioeconomic factors. Socioeconomic status is difficult to analyze. It also tends to denote life-style, amount of stress to which a person is subjected, general health status, and outlook. There is no clear indication that lower socioeconomic status leads to hypertension or increased cardiovascular mortality.

Increased heart rate. Increased heart rate with the same elevation in blood pressure is more likely to be associated with sudden death than lower heart rate.

Plasma renin. Hypertensives with high plasma renin activity show increased complications. However, evidence that plasma renin is responsible for any of these complications is nonconclusive.

EFFECT OF ARTERIAL PRESSURE ON LIFE EXPECTANCY AND MORTALITY

Virtually all the information about life expectancy and mortality in hypertension is derived from the experience of insurance companies. Elevated blood pressure of 150/100 mm. Hg at 45 years of age reduces the life expectancy by 8½ years in women and 11½ years in men. The same blood pressure in men at age 35 reduces life expectancy by 16½ years (from 41½ to 25 years).

It is now obvious, from the Build and Blood Pressure Study of the Society of Actuaries reported in 1959,[1] that the higher the arterial pressure when initially measured the greater the mortality. This is true from the lowest to the highest pressures, the relationship being quantitative. The most striking findings were that in men under 40 years of age a casual blood pressure of 140/90 mm. Hg is associated with an extra mortality of about 75%, whereas in men 40 years of age and older it is associated with an extra mortality of about 45%. In women the corresponding figures are 50% and 25%, respectively. The excess mortality associated with hypertension is chiefly due to cardiovascular and cerebrovascular diseases.

ECONOMIC CONSIDERATIONS OF HYPERTENSION CONTROL

Hypertension ranks as the number one public health problem of our time. For every employee killed by an industrial accident or industrial disease, more than 50 individuals die of cardiovascular diseases, with hypertension as the primary factor behind these. According to the American Heart Association's estimates of the cost of cardiovascular diseases in 1976, $9.3 billion were lost in wages, $2.8 billion were spent on physician and nursing services, $8.7 billion on hospital and nursing home service, and $0.8 billion on medications. Thus hypertension and cardiovascular diseases cost the nation over $20 billion in 1976. The unnecessary human suffering is inestimable.

Looking at the cost-effectiveness of hypertension control from society's point of view, Weinstein and Stason[8] believe that efforts to improve long-term follow-up care and medication adherence should receive priority. In their opinion, mass hypertension screening programs will be cost-effective only if adequate resources are available to ensure that detection is translated into effective long-term blood pressure control.

EFFECTS OF ANTIHYPERTENSIVE TREATMENT

The therapeutic effects that can be obtained with antihypertensive medications are illustrated by the data from the Veterans Administration Study Group[6,7] on antihypertensive agents. Antihypertensive therapy was 95% effective in preventing morbid events (e.g., congestive heart failure, myocardial infarction, cerebrovascular accidents) in men with diastolic blood pressure between 115 and 129 mm. Hg. In the group with 90 to 114 mm. Hg diastolic blood pressure, the treatment was demonstrated to be most effective in those with diastolic blood pressure above 104 mm. Hg. The Public Health Service data[5] demonstrate that the efficacy of treatment in women and in patients with diastolic blood pressure between 90 to 104 mm. Hg is not as great. However, if other risk factors are present, hypertension should be treated.

HYPERTENSION CONTROL IN CHILDREN

The National Heart, Lung and Blood Institute's Task Force on Blood Pressure Control in Children[4] made the following recommendations:

1. Children 3 years of age and older should have their blood pressure measured annually as part of their continuing health care.
2. Hypertension detection should be incorporated into the child's total health care program; high blood pressure detection programs per se for children should not be established. Referral and follow-up resources must be identified before detection activities begin.
3. Blood pressure measurements on infants and children should be taken in a quiet environment, with the correct cuff size and phase IV Korotkoff sound used for the diastolic pressure.
4. Blood pressure measurements obtained should be recorded on appropriate blood pressure charts.
5. Caution should be exercised in labeling children as "hypertensive" because of psychosocial and economic implications; use of the term "high normal blood pressure" is appropriate during evaluation and follow-up to avoid unnecessary negative implications.
6. Sustained blood pressure levels (obtained at least on three separate occasions) that are above the ninety-fifth percentile should be considered abnormal, with recognition that any cutoff point represents an arbitrary decision at any age.
7. In infants and children with sustained blood pressure above the ninety-fifth percentile, a medical history should be obtained, a physical examination performed, and further tests completed to determine a possible cause and to develop an appropriate follow-up program.
8. Children with sustained elevated blood pressure should receive a systematic long-term follow-up program, which may include hygienic counseling covering weight control, salt intake, exercise, and smoking and antihypertensive pharmacotherapy when indicated.
9. Physicians who manage hypertensive children with pharmacotherapy should use the "stepped-care" approach, with emphasis on minimal effective dosages of appropriate agents.
10. Children at high risk of developing elevated blood pressure should be evaluated for other atherosclerotic risk factors and should be taught to observe necessary hygienic measures for lowering risk factors.
11. Nurses and other properly trained and supervised nonphysician health personnel should participate in the identification and management of children with elevated blood pressure.

12. Specific research in the field of blood pressure control in children should be encouraged and funded. For this purpose, guidelines for research in children should be developed, including the evaluation of new drugs and other methods of blood pressure control.*

WHY HAVE WE FAILED?

Major reasons for uncontrolled hypertension include the asymptomatic nature of the condition, disagreement among physicians as to what constitutes hypertension, disagreement about the level of blood pressure at which treatment should be initiated, and the unpleasant side effects from medications decreasing patient compliance. In addition, patients discontinue medications because they "feel good" and do not see the need to continue the drug therapy. Successful communication between physician and patient focusing on the importance of sustained long-term therapy for hypertension must be established. The physician and nurse must be knowledgeable about optimal therapeutic regimens. In any medical care program for chronic disease, good long-term sustained therapy can and must be systematically assured by a combination of efforts involving both individual health care professionals working with individual patients and supplementary resources generated and organized by the community. This is necessary for continued success not only to control hypertension by modern pharmacologic means but also to achieve long-term adherence to such goals as cessation of cigarette smoking, appropriate diet, and weight control.

A TIME FOR ACTION

The National High Blood Pressure Education Program was organized in 1972. Its goals are to reduce the morbidity and mortality resulting from hypertension by enhancing professional and public awareness that hypertension is a real threat, its detection is important, and its treatment can reduce morbidity and mortality. The American people are being asked to have their blood pressure checked. By means of articles in national magazines and newspapers and television and radio advertisements, the public is being made aware of the need for detection and control of hypertension. However, health education is most convincing when information is given by one person to another, such as a physician or nurse to a patient and a parent or a teacher to a child.

This major chronic health problem presents us with important challenges. The physician may more effectively use his valuable time by concentrating efforts on the more serious complications of hypertension. Standardized treatment protocols can be effectively utilized by the nurse to manage mild and moderate hypertensives and to monitor well-controlled severe hypertensives. It is already becoming obvious that many nurse-managed clinics are performing excellent services for hypertension control. This new system provides the physician the

---

*From Report of the National Heart, Lung and Blood Institute's Task Force on Blood Pressure Control in Children, Pediatrics **59**:797-820, 1977.

opportunity and the satisfaction of providing the kind of medical care that can literally help millions of people enjoy extra years of living. No government agency or professional association can do this job alone. Hypertension control can only be accomplished through a team effort in which the physician, as the team leader, delegates authority and shares the responsibility with the nurse and allied health care professionals in caring for hypertensive patients.

Emerson said, "This time, like all times, is a very good one if we know what to do with it." Fortunately we know what to do in this instance. We have to control hypertension. The time for action is now.

SUMMARY

Hypertension is defined as blood pressure of 160/95 mm. Hg or above. Blood pressure below 140/90 mm. Hg is considered normal for adults. Between these two levels, hypertension is considered borderline. Almost 25% of the population have persistent hypertension, and 10% have labile hypertension. The complications of hypertension can be divided into those which are specifically related to the hypertension and those which are due to the accompanying atherosclerosis. Hypertensive complications include malignant hypertension, cerebral hemorrhage, congestive heart failure, and dissecting aortic aneurysm. Certain conditions or situations increase the propensity to atherosclerosis. These risk factors include hypertension, old age, male sex, elevated serum cholesterol, black race, cigarette smoking, diabetes, heredity, obesity, excessive alcohol consumption, sedentary life-style, increased heart rate, and elevated plasma renin.

✓ Hypertension reduces life expectancy, and the higher the pressure the greater the mortality. The adverse economic impact of hypertension and cardiovascular diseases is enormous. Treatment of hypertension helps reduce morbidity and mortality from the hypertensive complications, whereas the effect of treatment on atherosclerotic complications is not as readily apparent. Although control of hypertension can be achieved with relative ease, a large majority of hypertensives remain undetected, untreated, or uncontrolled. These people urgently need their hypertension detected, evaluated, and controlled.

SUGGESTED READINGS

1. Build and Blood Pressure Study, 1959, vols. 1 and 2, 1959, Society of Actuaries.
2. Friedman, M.: The psychological profile of the hypertensive patient: an explanation of his therapeutic response, Bulletin No. 50008A, New York, 1975, American Heart Association.
3. Kannel, W. B., McGee, D., and Gordon, T.: A general cardiovascular risk profile: the Framingham study, Am. J. Cardiol. **38:**46-51, 1976.
4. Report of the National Heart, Lung and Blood Institute's Task Force on Blood Pressure Control in Children, Pediatrics **59:**797-820, 1977.
5. Smith, W. M. (Chairman), U.S. Public Health Service Hospitals Cooperative Study Group: Treatment of mild hypertension—results of a 10-year intervention trial, Circ. Res. **40**(supp. 1):98-105, 1977.
6. Veterans Administration Cooperative Study Group on Antihypertensive Agents: Effects of treatment on morbidity in hypertension. I. Results in patients with diastolic blood pressure averaging 115 through 129 mm. Hg, J.A.M.A. **202:**1028-1034, 1967.

7. Veterans Administration Cooperative Study Group on Antihypertensive Agents: Effects of treatment on morbidity in hypertension. II. Results in patients with diastolic blood pressure averaging 90 through 114 mm. Hg, J.A.M.A. **213:**1143-1152, 1970.

8. Weinstein, M. C., and Stason, W. B.: Hypertension: a policy perspective, Cambridge, 1976, Harvard University Press.

CHAPTER 2

Blood pressure regulation and pathophysiology of hypertension

Blood pressure is the lateral pressure exerted by a column of blood on the vessel wall. The term "blood pressure," or "BP," implies the systemic arterial pressure.

NORMAL REGULATION OF BLOOD PRESSURE

Many factors and organ systems are responsible for the normal regulation of blood pressure. The major factors involved are cardiac output, peripheral resistance, blood volume, and blood viscosity. The organs that are involved include the sympathetic nervous system, kidneys, and adrenals. A description of their respective roles follows.

Cardiac output

Cardiac output is the volume of blood ejected by the left ventricle into the aorta per minute. It is the major determining factor of the systolic blood pressure. The cardiac output is a function of the heart rate and stroke volume. Stroke vol-

14

ume is the amount of blood ejected from the heart each beat. In situations such as exercise when the heart rate rises, as long as the stroke volume remains unchanged, the cardiac output increases. This causes the systolic blood pressure to rise. After the heart rate rises above a certain rate, usually more than 150 beats/min., the ventricular filling is incomplete, and the stroke volume diminishes, causing a fall in cardiac output and systolic blood pressure. As the left ventricle ejects blood, the aorta relaxes to accommodate it, thus playing a modulating role. If the aorta is rigid because of atherosclerosis, as happens in elderly patients, it is unable to exert this modulating effect, causing systolic hypertension.

Peripheral resistance

The diastolic blood pressure is primarily determined by the resistance in the arterioles, which is a function of the muscular tone in the media of the arteriolar wall. Arterioles constitute the distal-most segment of the arterial system. Their average diameter is about 1 mm. The arterioles have a rich supply of the sympathetic nerves. Norepinephrine released from these adrenergic nerve endings acts on the smooth muscle cells, causing vasoconstriction.

Blood volume

Blood volume is also an important determinant of the blood pressure. In instances in which there is acute hemorrhage or loss of plasma volume as may happen in patients with severe burns, blood volume suddenly diminishes and the blood pressure falls, resulting in a state of cardiovascular shock. On the other hand, rapid expansion of blood volume with intravenous fluids causes the blood pressure to rise.

Blood viscosity

Blood viscosity is the internal friction of molecules against each other. Relative to water, plasma has a viscosity of about 1.5 and whole blood, about 4.0. In conditions such as polycythemia in which the number of red cells in the blood is increased or in hypergammaglobulinemias such as multiple myeloma and Waldenström's macroglobulinemia, the viscosity of blood is enhanced, causing subsequent elevation in blood pressure.

Sympathetic nervous activity

Sympathetic nervous activity plays a prominent role in regulation of blood pressure. Increased sympathetic activity as may occur in fear, flight, or fight situations leads to increased secretion of catecholamines (adrenalin and noradrenalin), which cause elevation in blood pressure. On standing suddenly from the supine position, the blood tends to accumulate in the lower extremities. The sympathetic tone immediately rises, causing vasoconstriction, which not only prevents the fall in blood pressure but causes it to rise by 5 to 10 mm. Hg. Because of sympathetic insufficiency, in patients with postural hypotension, the blood pressure drops on standing, causing orthostatic symptoms of dizziness and fainting.

Kidneys

The kidney plays an extremely significant role in the regulation of blood pressure. It is largely responsible for maintenance of the fluid and electrolyte balance of the body. In conditions in which the plasma volume is constricted, the kidney can absorb almost all the sodium that is filtered in an attempt to expand the plasma volume. In addition, it secretes an enzyme called "renin." Renin is produced in the juxtaglomerular apparatus, which is comprised of hypertrophied smooth muscle cells of the afferent arteriole and a segment of the corresponding distal tubule, the macula densa. The output of renin is increased by sodium depletion, hypovolemia, stimulation of sympathetic nerves, secretion of catecholamines, adoption of the upright posture, and drugs such as diuretics and vasodilator antihypertensives. Alterations in tubular fluid composition and vascular stretch also stimulate renin secretion. It is decreased by the administration of mineralocorticoids or β blockers. In the blood circulation, renin acts on an α_2 globulin called "renin substrate," or "angiotensinogen," to produce angiotensin I. Angiotensin I is further split by a converting enzyme mainly in lung capillaries to form the active angiotensin II, which is a potent vasoconstrictor. Angiotensin II and its metabolite, angiotensin III, stimulate the adrenal to produce aldosterone. Angiotensin II is rapidly inactivated by peptidase enzymes, angiotensinases, in the blood, and therefore constant synthesis is required for lasting effect.

Adrenals

The adrenal cortical and medullary hormones play major roles in the regulation of blood pressure. The mineralocorticoid, aldosterone, produced in the zona glomerulosa, the outer layer of the adrenal cortex, is the most important mineralocorticoid hormone. As previously indicated, aldosterone secretion is stimulated by angiotensin II. It is also secreted in response to hyperkalemia and adrenocorticotropic hormone (ACTH). Aldosterone acts primarily at the distal tubule and the collecting duct of the nephron. It enhances sodium absorption and potassium excretion at this site. Sodium retention leads to expansion of extracellular volume and elevation in blood pressure. 11-Deoxycorticosterone (DOC), another mineralocorticoid, is also secreted at the same rate as aldosterone. However, it has only about a thirtieth of the mineralocorticoid potency of aldosterone and therefore is of little physiologic importance. Cortisol is the major hormone secreted by the adrenal cortex. It has many metabolic functions in the body and some mineralocorticoid effect. Its secretion is primarily controlled by ACTH.

The adrenal medulla is the major site of adrenalin secretion. Generally, the noradrenalin secreted at the peripheral nerve endings is responsible for sympathetic control of blood pressure. However, as indicated before, in emergency situations of fear, flight, or fight, adrenalin is released into the circulation, causing elevation in blood pressure.

Autacoids (vasoactive substances)

Autacoids include the noncirculating tissue hormones prostaglandins and kinins. The prostaglandins are 20-carbon unsaturated fatty acids. There are four major families of prostaglandins: A, E, F, and I. Lee has postulated that in the absence of prostaglandins, vasoconstriction would lead to increased peripheral resistance and elevation in blood pressure. Itskovitz and McGiff have demonstrated prostaglandins to be vasodilators in the kidney. They are found to inhibit the renal pressor mechanisms such as the renin/angiotensin system.

Kinins are vasodilator peptides produced primarily in the kidney and are thought to exert a modulating action on blood pressure. Their exact role remains to be defined.

Maintenance of normal blood pressure

Under normal circumstances, the blood pressure level is maintained by interplay of the various mechanisms just described. Alterations in sympathetic nervous activity by affecting the cardiac output and the peripheral resistance help overcome a sudden fall or rise in blood pressure. The renal and adrenal cortical mechanisms, on the other hand, help in the long-range maintenance of normal blood pressure.

PATHOPHYSIOLOGY OF ESSENTIAL HYPERTENSION[1]

As indicated in Chapter 1, more than 90% of patients with elevated blood pressure do not have an identifiable disease as a cause of their hypertension. These patients are said to have "essential (idiopathic, primary) hypertension." Although these patients do not have an identifiable cause for their hypertension, the following alterations in their blood pressure regulation mechanisms have been identified. Whether these alterations are the cause or the result of hypertension is not always clear.

Increased cardiac output and peripheral resistance

In the overwhelming majority of studies, patients with established although mild hypertension show a normal cardiac output and increased peripheral resistance. However, several investigators have identified a group of hypertensives who have an increased cardiac output as the major hemodynamic abnormality with normal peripheral resistance. Most of these patients were early hypertensives with a hyperkinetic circulation, a rapid pulse rate, and frequently labile hypertension. It has been proposed that an increased cardiac output occurs at the onset of hypertension, but adjustments are made by the body which bring the blood pressure back to normal while the peripheral resistance increases. The peripheral vascular bed probably has the ability to regulate the flow of blood, depending on the metabolic need of tissues; the vessels contract and the blood flow decreases. Peripheral resistance increases and blood pressure rises further. This activates the baroreceptors, which bring about a normalization of the cardiac output through a reflex mechanism. Patients have been described who have been shown to progress from an initial high-output, normal resistance state to a normal-output, high resistance state. In a few situations increased cardiac output definitely plays an important role in raising the arterial pressure. These are renal failure, toxemia of pregnancy, thyrotoxicosis, and acute glomerulonephritis.

Retention of salt and water

Salt and extracellular fluid volume excess also play a significant role in both the genesis and perpetration of human hypertension. Guyton believes that in many essential hypertensives, early in the course of the disease, the kidney is unable to excrete salt and water in a normal fashion. Under normal circumstances, when arterial pressure rises, urinary output of salt and water increases shrinking fluid volume until arterial pressure falls back to normal. In essential hypertension, there must be renal dysfunction. Thus in the face of elevated blood pressure, the kidney is unable to increase output of salt and water, resulting in a new steady state with normal body fluid volume, normal cardiac output, and normal renal excretion of salt and water at the cost of elevated arterial blood pressure.

Excessive salt intake is considered responsible for initiation of essential hypertension in many individuals. Dahl and colleagues demonstrated that there are salt-sensitive and salt-insensitive strains of rats, so that a distinct possibility exists of a genetic factor acting in conjunction with high salt intake to produce hypertension. Population studies of salt intake have demonstrated that the Solomon Island natives, who eat little salt in their diet, do not develop elevation in blood pressure with advancing age. However, natives of an offshore island, who cook their fish in the ocean water containing 3% salt, develop hypertension at an extremely early age. It has been proposed that "soul foods" with their high-salt content play a major role in causing hypertension among blacks in the United States.

The sodium chloride content of arteriolar cells is increased in hypertension. This causes swelling, "water-logging," and thickening of the arteriolar wall, which increases the vascular reactivity and peripheral resistance, further elevating the blood pressure.

Low-salt intake and treatment with diuretics reduce extracellular volume and intracellular sodium chloride, thus helping reduce blood pressure.

Altered renin/angiotensin/aldosterone balance

Although in most patients with essential hypertension the plasma renin level is normal, in almost 15% of patients the plasma renin is inappropriately elevated. These have been classified as "high-renin essential hypertensives."

Some investigators have found an increase of circulating angiotensin II, the most potent vasoconstrictor known, in these hypertensives. Elevated aldosterone level has also been reported in certain essential hypertensives. It is thus possible that inappropriate renin/angiotensin/aldosterone activity may be responsible for hypertension in at least a few patients with essential hypertension.

Excessive mineralocorticoids

Certain investigators believe that patients with essential hypertension have elevated levels of mineralocorticoids other than aldosterone. Almost 25% of patients with essential hypertension have low-renin hypertension. It is possible that these patients have excessive unidentifiable circulating mineralocorticoids which are able to suppress renin secretion and cause hypertension. These hormones are probably secreted from the adrenal gland and are chemically related to DOC.

Stress and increased sympathetic activity

Physiologic responses to stress, which are normally protective and adaptive, may persist to a pathologic degree possibly as a result of learned behavior patterns, resulting in excessive hypothalamic discharge and increased sympathetic nervous activity. Several investigators have demonstrated elevated plasma norepinephrine and catecholamine excretion in the urine in certain essential hypertensive patients. Clinical and hemodynamic evidence exists implicating sympathetic nervous dysfunction in hypertension.

Secondary mechanisms may develop in hypertensive patients with a primary neurogenic stimulus, which then may serve to accelerate the hypertension. Since norepinephrine is a stimulus for renin release, increased sympathetic nervous activity may result in increased angiotensin II, which may further result in vasoconstriction and increased aldosterone secretion, all leading to elevated blood pressure. Under normal circumstances, the sympathetic nervous activity is reversed by the reuptake of norepinephrine into sympathetic nerve endings. It is possible that in certain hypertensives, sympathetic nerve defects exist that decrease norepinephrine uptake and storage capacity.

The fact that sympathetic inhibitors are the mainstay of treatment of hypertension leads one to the logical conclusion that the sympathetic nervous system plays an important role in pathogenesis and perpetuation of the hypertensive state.

Lack of vasodilator substances

It has been proposed that deficiency of prostglandins, kinins, and other vasodilators may be responsible for essential hypertension.

Volume vasoconstriction hypothesis

According to Laragh,[2] vasoconstriction and volume excess are the two determining factors in essential hypertension (Fig. 4). He believes that either vasoconstriction or excessive blood volume is responsible for elevated blood pressure

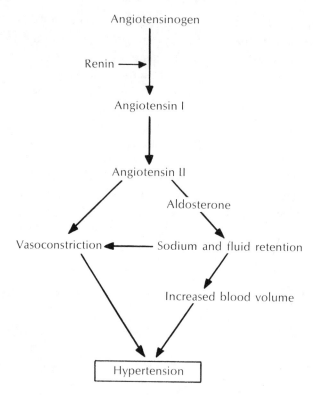

Fig. 4. Volume vasoconstriction hypothesis of essential hypertension.

in the majority of hypertensives. Those that do not fall into these extreme categories have various combinations of vasoconstriction and volume excess. Patients with a primarily vasoconstriction state have high plasma renin activity, and those with volume excess have low plasma renin activity.

Although the hypothesis is attractive and may explain some of the final steps in the long process that leads to essential hypertension, it does not answer the basic question as to what triggers the initial elevation in blood pressure and why it is sustained despite numerous regulatory mechanisms that normally tend to normalize the blood pressure.

Hypertension as multifactorial disorder

The Mosaic theory first proposed by Page in 1949 takes all the abnormalities first described into account and considers hypertension the end result of abnormalities in blood pressure regulation. Fig. 5 summarizes how one or more factors may initiate a process that ultimately results in hypertension.

PATHOPHYSIOLOGY OF SECONDARY HYPERTENSION[3]

Although the majority of hypertensives have essential hypertension, a significant minority (approximately 5%) have secondary hypertension. This is more

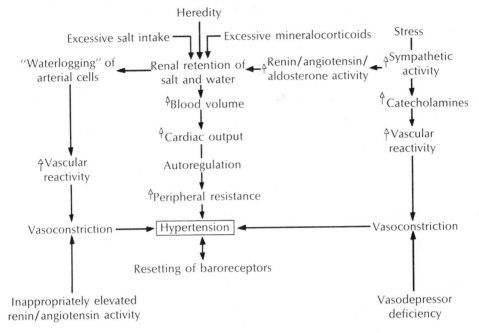

Fig. 5. Essential hypertension as a multifactorial disorder.

common in children. In children, severe hypertension is almost always secondary in nature. Following is a discussion of the common causes of hypertension and the mechanisms in these situations.

Renal hypertension

Among the many renal diseases known to be associated with hypertension, the important examples include acute and chronic glomerulonephritis, polycystic disease of the kidney, diabetic kidney disease, polyarteritis nodosa, chronic pyelonephritis, hemangiopericytoma (renin-producing tumor), and renal trauma.

The exact mechanism of hypertension in these renal disorders is not always clear. Fluid retention may be responsible in patients with end-stage kidney disease. This is called "renoprival hypertension." Dialysis and removal of excessive fluid often reduce blood pressure. In many such cases, plasma renin is elevated and the renin/angiotensin/aldosterone system may be responsible for hypertension. In a few cases of end-stage renal disease, hypertension is present despite normal blood volume and normal plasma renin activity.

In patients with early renal disease in which there is no fluid retention or elevated plasma renin activity, the mechanism of hypertension frequently is unclear. In these situations, hypertension may be a result of accumulation of certain vasopressor substances that are normally metabolized and excreted by the kidney or a result of the inability of the diseased kidney to generate certain vasodilator substances like the prostaglandins and kinins.

Renal artery stenosis

Constriction of one or both renal arteries, as may happen in congenital fibromuscular hyperplasia or atherosclerotic narrowing of the renal arteries, often results in hypertension.

Fibromuscular hyperplasia (also called "fibrous dysplasia") is more common in white women under the age of 50 years. A family history of hypertension is usually absent. A continuous upper abdominal bruit is often present. Pathologically the fibrotic lesions have been classified on the basis of their location within the renal artery. Intimal fibroplasia, medial hyperplasia, intimal fibroplasia with microaneurysms, medial dissection, perimedial fibroplasia, and periadventitial fibroplasia have been described. Clinically these pathologic lesions seem to be of little significance. The resulting ischemia of the renal tissue leads to excessive renin secretion and activation of the renin/angiotensin/aldosterone system, which leads to elevated blood pressure. Resection of the stenotic lesion or its bypass with reestablishment of normal renal blood flow frequently results in cure of hypertension. However, the disease generally is progressive and can also involve other arteries such as the splenic and hepatic arteries.

Renal artery stenosis due to atherosclerosis usually occurs in patients over 50 years of age. The lesion is an atherosclerotic plaque most frequently present at the origin of the renal artery. On angiography the abdominal aorta often shows extensive irregularity because of atherosclerosis. These patients have a shorter duration of hypertension, are more likely to have exudative and hemorrhagic retinopathy, and have a higher frequency of upper abdominal bruits. Most of these patients have essential hypertension to start with, which may become more severe because of renal ischemia secondary to renal artery stenosis. Renal ischemia may also result from extraneous pressure on the renal artery as may occur with a tumor or a congenital fibrous band.

Primary aldosteronism

Generally, primary aldosteronism is caused by an aldosterone-secreting adenoma (Conn's syndrome), but occasionally it is associated with adrenal hyperplasia or with morphologically normal adrenal glands (idiopathic hyperaldosteronism). Primary aldosteronism is responsible for hypertension in less than 1% of the hypertensive population. It is twice as common in females as males and is rare in blacks.

Usually aldosterone promotes the conservation of sodium and the excretion of potassium. Hypersecretion of aldosterone therefore leads to excessive loss of potassium in the urine and hypokalemia, causing muscular weakness, fatigue, areflexia, tetany, paresthesias, certain electrocardiographic abnormalities, and impaired concentration of the urine by the kidney leading to polyuria and nocturia. Excessive conservation of sodium initially leads to expansion of extracellular volume and elevation of the blood pressure. The blood pressure remains elevated during the course of the disease. However, progressive expansion of extracellular volume is avoided by certain physiologic adjustments. This is termed the "escape phenomenon."

Secondary aldosteronism as compared to primary aldosteronism is not a disease but a response of the normal adrenal gland to excessive renin secretion, as may be seen in conditions such as dehydration, hemorrhage, hypoalbuminemic states, congestive heart failure, nephrotic syndrome, and hepatic cirrhosis. This does not usually cause hypertension; however, hypokalemia may be a prominent feature.

Cushing's syndrome

Cushing's syndrome is the clinical and metabolic disorder resulting from a chronic excess production of cortisol (hydrocortisone). There are three well-established causes of Cushing's syndrome:

1. *Adrenocortical tumors.* These can be carcinomas, solitary adenomas, or (rarely) multiple adenomas.

2. *Ectopic ACTH syndrome.* Certain nonpituitary malignant neoplasms secrete ACTH, which stimulates the adrenal cortex to secrete excessive amounts of cortisol, causing clinical Cushing's syndrome.

3. *Cushing's disease.* Excessive ACTH production by the pituitary usually due to a basophil or a chromophobe adenoma leads to stimulation of the adrenal gland and excessive cortisol production.

Cortisol has several important metabolic functions but, in addition, has mineralocorticoid action similar to aldosterone. Therefore it promotes potassium excretion and sodium retention, causing hypertension and hypokalemia. Clinical features of Cushing's syndrome include central obesity, rounding of the face, prominent abdominal striae, and hirsutism. Additional abnormalities may include impaired glucose tolerance, osteoporosis, muscular atrophy, edema, kidney stones, and psychotic mentation.

Pheochromocytoma

Pheochromocytoma is a catecholamine-producing tumor arising from the cells of the sympathetic nervous system. The tumor is usually located in the adrenal gland but can occur in the paravertebral sympathetic ganglia. Most patients have a single benign pheochromocytoma. Malignant tumors are found in fewer than 10% of patients. Pheochromocytomas can be inherited in association with medullary carcinoma of the thyroid and a tendency to parathyroid hyperfunction resulting from hyperplasia or multiple parathyroid adenomas (Sipple's syndrome). Multiple neurofibromata and café au lait spots on the skin may be present in some patients.

The hypertension is due to excessive production of catecholamines and is classically paroxysmal in character. It is often associated with palpitations, tachycardia, a feeling of malaise, apprehension, and excessive sweating. Many patients are persistently hypertensive, having superimposed paroxysmal rises in blood pressure. The paroxysm may be precipitated by emotional upset, postural change, physical exertion, and sometimes eating. Blood pressure recorded during severe attacks may exceed 300 mm. Hg and leave the patient weak and tired. In addition to hypertension and the paroxysmal symptoms just described, these patients have orthostatic hypotension, polycythemia, impaired glucose tolerance, and constipation. Increased incidence of cholelithiasis has been noted in patients with pheochromocytoma.

Coarctation of the aorta

Coarctation of the aorta is a narrowing of the aortic lumen due to a localized deformity of the vascular media and a curtainlike infolding. It is characteristically located distal to the origin of the left subclavian artery but can occasionally occur proximal to the orifice of that vessel. This condition predominately occurs in males and is often associated with a bicuspid aortic valve and an aneurysm of the circle of Willis. The patient may complain of headache, spontaneous epistaxis, and leg fatigue. Hypertension in the upper extremities and low or normal blood pressure in the lower extremities is the hallmark of this condition. The femoral pulses are usually feeble and definitely delayed. Collateral arteries may be seen on the patient's back.

The renin secretion is high because of compromised renal blood flow. Excessive renin secretion triggers angiotensin II and aldosterone production, which contributes to the patient's hypertension. Surgical correction of the coarctation, if done at an early age, corrects the hypertension. However, postoperative hypertension and increased cardiovascular disease have been described on long-term follow-up of these patients.

Toxemia of pregnancy

Toxemia occurs late in pregnancy and is characterized by hypertension, edema, and proteinuria. It is called "preeclampsia" in absence of convulsions and "eclampsia" when they are present. Presence of convulsions is usually indicative of severe disease. Toxemia is more common with preexisting renal disease, hypertension, and diabetes, with twin pregnancies, and in black women.

Usually the blood pressure falls during early pregnancy. A simple "rollover" test done about the twenty-fourth week of pregnancy may help predict the occurrence of toxemia later in pregnancy. This test is performed by recording the blood pressure after having the patient lie on her left side for about 20 minutes. She then rolls over and lies on her back. A rise of 20 to 25 mm. Hg systolic or 10 to 15 mm. Hg diastolic blood pressure is considered a positive "rollover" test.

The mechanism of hypertension in toxemia of pregnancy is unclear. Salt retention caused by the reduction in glomerular filtration rate, renin production by the placenta because of ischemia, and increased sensitivity to angiotensin seem to play a role in causing toxemia and the accompanying hypertension. Although plasma renin levels are normal, they are considered inappropriately high in the face of fluid retention and hypertension. The role of prostaglandins has been much speculated but is still unsettled in the pathogenesis of toxemia.

Medication-induced hypertension

Oral contraceptives and *estrogen preparations* are a well-known cause of medication-induced hypertension. Between 5% and 7% of women receiving oral contraceptives develop hypertension requiring discontinuation of medication. Although the exact mechanism of hypertension in this situation is unknown, oral contraceptives stimulate production of renin substrate (angiotensinogen) from the liver. This may lead to excessive production of angiotensin and aldosterone, causing hypertension. However, women receiving oral contraceptives who do not develop hypertension also have increased renin substrate production. It has been postulated that patients who develop hypertension do not metabolize angiotensin as efficiently as those who do not develop hypertension. Discontinuation of oral contraceptive therapy usually leads to reversal of hypertension within 6 months.

Corticosteroids (hydrocortisone, prednisone, and analogues) are the most commonly used drugs that are responsible for iatrogenic hypertension. Large pharmacologic doses of corticosteroids are used in management of bronchial asthma, allergies, collagen vascular disorders, skin diseases, kidney diseases such as glomerulonephritis, and after renal transplantation and many other disorders. Hypertension is, as in Cushing's syndrome, due to salt and water retention.

Sympathetic stimulators such as amphetamines and analogues used for appetite suppression and ephedrine and analogues used for asthma and nasal congestion produce vasoconstriction and therefore hypertension. Amphetamine is now rarely clinically prescribed but is a widely abused drug. It has been reported to produce vasculitis in the kidney and thus can produce hypertension through renal mechanisms as well.

Licorice, present in black candy and certain medications used for peptic ulcer treatment in Europe, contains glycerrhizic acid, which has a mineralocorticoid effect causing salt and water retention.

Miscellaneous conditions causing hypertension

Certain *ovarian tumors* may cause overproduction of steroid hormones and lead to hypertension in a way similar to Cushing's syndrome. *Cerebral hemorrhage* and *intracranial neoplasms* may increase intracranial tension acutely and cause hypertension through alterations in a centrally located blood pressure control mechanism. Administration of *monoamine oxidase inhibitor drugs followed by tyramine* contained in foods and beverages such as cheese, beer, and pickles may cause acute elevation in blood pressure through accumulation of norepinephrine in the blood.

SUMMARY

The term "blood pressure" (BP) implies systemic arterial pressure. Normal blood pressure is a function of cardiac output, peripheral resistance, blood volume, and blood viscosity. The sympathetic nervous system by means of neurohumors, adrenalin, and noradrenalin, regulates blood pressure from minute to minute. The kidneys and adrenals by means of the renin/angiotensin/aldosterone system are responsible for the long-range maintenance of normal blood pressure.

Although the definite cause and pathogenesis of essential hypertension are not known, several abnormalities in blood pressure regulation have been identified. Heredity and environmental stress seem to play key roles in initiating the process. Altered kidney function causing salt and water retention, renin/angiotensin/aldosterone imbalance, and increased sympathetic activity have been implicated in perpetration of elevated blood pressure.

Secondary hypertension results from various renal, adrenal, and vascular abnormalities. Frequently, hypertension can be surgically cured in these situations. Although the anatomic lesion can be identified, the mechanism of hypertension is not always clear, and even after surgery mild hypertension may persist requiring medical therapy.

Medication-induced hypertension is not uncommon. The most common cause of hypertension in white women under the age of 45 years is intake of oral contraceptive pills.

SUGGESTED READINGS

1. Laragh, J. H.: Hypertension manual, New York, 1973, Dun-Donnelley.
2. Laragh, J. H.: Modern system for treating high blood pressure based on renin profiling and vaso-constriction-volume analysis: a primary role for beta blocking drugs such as propranolol, Am. J. Med. **61:**797-810, 1976.
3. Onesti, G., Kim, K. E., and Moyer, J. H.: Hypertension: mechanisms and management, Twenty-Sixth Hahnemann Symposium, New York, 1973, Grune & Stratton, Inc.

CHAPTER 3

Clinical pharmacology of antihypertensive drugs

Drugs play an important role in the management of hypertension. Life-style modifications are usually insufficient to control hypertension in most patients. With the use of modern antihypertensive drugs, blood pressure can be normalized in almost all patients with essential hypertension and in certain patients with secondary hypertension. Since secondary hypertension can often be cured surgically, the drug treatment is usually reserved for patients with essential hypertension.

HISTORY AND RATIONALE

Low-salt diet and surgical sympathectomy were used as treatment of hypertension in the first half of the twentieth century. The antihypertensive effect of reserpine was demonstrated in the late forties, and it became the drug of choice for treatment of hypertension about 1950. Veratrum alkaloids and ganglion-blocking drugs were also used as antihypertensive agents but were found to have unacceptable side effects. Thiazide diuretics were introduced in 1957, and their antihypertensive potential became evident a year later. Since then they have been used increasingly for the treatment of essential hypertension and are now the drug of first choice. Methyldopa (Aldomet), a sympathetic inhibitor, has been used in the treatment of hypertension since 1962. Several other agents have been introduced since then. Certain drugs have proved more useful than others in lowering blood pressure. Almost all antihypertensives have side effects, some more than others.

The drug treatment of hypertension acquired firm footing on the basis of the Veterans Administration Cooperative Study, which used a thiazide diuretic in conjunction with reserpine and hydralazine for the control of hypertension. The results of this study have been discussed in Chapter 1. Although similar results have not been demonstrated using other modern antihypertensive drugs, it is assumed that the salutary effects of the drugs used in the Veterans Administration study were due to their antihypertensive action. Therefore similar results can be expected using other drugs as long as the hypertension is controlled.

MODERN ANTIHYPERTENSIVE DRUGS[1,3]

Antihypertensive drugs presently used in the treatment of hypertension can be classified as follows on the basis of their site of action (Fig. 6).
I. Diuretics
    A. Thiazide and related diuretics
    B. Loop diuretics: furosemide and ethacrynic acid
    C. Potassium-sparing diuretics: spironolactone and triamterene

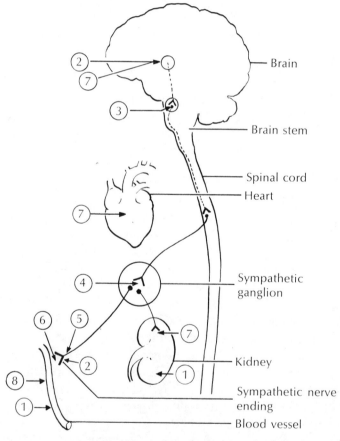

Fig. 6. Site of action of antihypertensive drugs. *1,* Diuretics; *2,* reserpine and methyldopa; *3,* clonidine; *4,* trimethaphan; *5,* guanethidine; *6,* phentolamine and phenoxybenzamine; *7,* propanolol; *8,* vasodilators.

II. Sympathetic inhibitors
    A. Centrally acting: reserpine, methyldopa, and clonidine
    B. Ganglion blockers: trimethaphan
    C. Adrenergic nerve ending blockers: guanethidine and reserpine
    D. Receptor blockers
        1. α blockers: phentolamine and phenoxybenzamine
        2. β blockers: propranolol
III. Vasodilators
    A. Hydralazine
    B. Prazosin
    C. Sodium nitroprusside
    D. Diazoxide

Diuretics

The diuretics are the mainstay of treatment of essential hypertension. Drug treatment of hypertension is initiated with a diuretic. Other antihypertensive drugs are added to the diuretic until the blood pressure is controlled. Table 1 lists the diuretics presently available for use in treatment of hypertension and Fig. 7 depicts their site of action in the nephron.

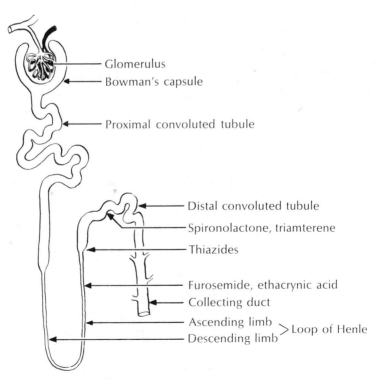

Fig. 7. Site of action of diuretics in the nephron.

Table 1. Diuretics presently in use

Generic name	Trade name	Size of tablets (mg.)	Dose range (mg./24 hr.)	Duration of action (hr.)
Thiazides and thiazide derivatives				
Chlorothiazide	Diuril	250 and 500	500-1000	6-12
Hydrochlorothiazide	Hydrodiuril, Esidrex, Oretic	25 and 50	50-100	6-12
Flumethiazide		500	500-1000	6-12
Benzthiazide	Exna	50	50-100	12-18
Hydroflumethiazide	Saluron	50	50-100	18-24
Bendroflumethiazide	Naturetin	2.5 and 5	2.5-5.0	18-24
Cyclothiazide	Anhydron	2	1.0-2.0	18-24
Methylclothiazide	Enduron	2.5 and 5	2.5-5.0	24+
Polythiazide	Renese	1, 2, and 4	1.0-4.0	24-36
Trichlormethiazide	Naqua, Metahydrin	2 and 4	2.0-4.0	24-36
Quinethazone	Hydromox	50	50-100	24-36
Chlorthalidone	Hygroton	50 and 100	50-100	48-72
Metolazone	Zaroxolyn	2.5, 5, and 10	2.5-10	48-72
Loop diuretics				
Furosemide	Lasix	20 and 40	20-160	4-6
Ethacrynic acid	Edecrin	25 and 50	25-200	4-6
Potassium-sparing diuretics				
Triamterene	Dyrenium	50 and 100	50-300	2-8
Spironolactone	Aldactone	25	25-200	12-48

Thiazide and related diuretics. Chlorothiazide and hydrochlorothiazide are the representative diuretics in this group. Many analogues are available and have similar properties. Although they differ from one another in terms of potency (the dose required to attain a desired effect), there is little difference in their efficacy (the maximum beneficial effect).

The thiazide diuretics are sulfonamide derivatives. As a group they are designated as benzothiadiazide compounds. Chlorthalidone, quinethazone, and metolazone differ somewhat chemically from the thiazides.

The dominant action of the thiazides is to increase the renal excretion of sodium chloride and water. A significant part of the antihypertensive action of diuretic agents is due to mild to moderate volume contraction. Possible direct vasodilator effect by reduction of sodium and chloride ions in the arteriolar smooth muscle cells may also play a role.

Thiazides decrease vascular reactivity, thus blunting the effectiveness of the sympathetic reflexes. Peripheral resistance is gradually lowered, causing both systolic and diastolic blood pressures to drop by 10 to 15 mm. Hg.

The thiazides are rapidly absorbed from the gastrointestinal tract. Most agents demonstrate diuretic effect within an hour. The thiazides are distributed throughout the extracellular space, readily cross the placental barrier, and are excreted in the mother's milk. Most compounds are rapidly excreted within 3 to 6 hours, although the long-acting diuretics are excreted slowly. Thiazides are excreted essentially unchanged in the urine. In the absence of renal function, they are excreted in the bile.

The thiazides are often sufficient in the treatment of mild hypertension but may be utilized in conjunction with other antihypertensives in the treatment of moderate and severe hypertension. They are also used in the treatment of congestive heart failure and diabetes insipidus. Hypersensitivity to thiazides or other sulfonamide-derived drugs is a contraindication to their use. The use of thiazides for treatment of edema in pregnancy is controversial; however, they can be used cautiously in the treatment of hypertension during pregnancy. It may be wise to avoid their use in the nursing mother.

The thiazides may produce hypokalemia, hyperuricemia, hyperglycemia, hypercalcemia, and hyperlipidemia. In a dose of hydrochlorothiazide equal to or less than 50 mg./24 hr., hypokalemia is usually mild, rarely symptomatic, and seldom necessitates addition of potassium supplement. Attention to potassium balance deserves emphasis in patients with heart disease, especially if they are taking digitalis, since the risk of developing cardiac arrhythmia in the presence of hypokalemia is substantial. Prevention of hypokalemia can generally be accomplished in the vast majority of patients by a high dietary intake of potassium.

Clinically, significant hyperuricemia rarely develops with chronic diuretic use. In the patient with gout, treatment with allopurinol (Zyloprim) or probenecid (Benemid) will usually allow continuation of the diuretic without recurrent symptoms. Hyperglycemia is not a major problem, and diabetes is not a contraindication to the use of diuretics in the treatment of hypertension. Dietary adjustment and appropriate pharmacologic treatment of diabetes can be carried out simultaneously. Hypercalcemia, although demonstrated biochemically, is seldom of any clinical significance. Hyperlipidemia has been reported recently with chronic use of diuretics. Elevation of triglyceride levels is usually more pronounced than cholesterol. The clinical significance of this side effect remains to be defined.

When used in pregnancy, fetal neonatal jaundice and thrombocytopenia have been reported.

Preparations and dosages are listed in Table 1.

Loop diuretics. The diuretics of this class include furosemide (Lasix) and ethacrynic acid (Edecrin). These drugs effect a peak diuresis far greater than that observed with thiazides by promptly inhibiting sodium and chloride transport in the ascending limb of the loop of Henle.

These drugs are the carboxylic acids of moderately complex compounds, having little in common structurally. Thus they constitute a pharmacologic rather than a chemical class.

They are readily absorbed from the gastrointestinal tract and are bound to plasma proteins considerably. After oral ingestion, the diuretic response begins within an hour and after intravenous injection, within 2 to 10 minutes. They are rapidly excreted in the urine by glomerular filtration and tubular secretion. Furosemide is excreted in the feces as well.

The mechanism of actions and effects on blood pressure are similar to those of thiazide diuretics.

The antihypertensive potential of loop diuretics is probably equivalent to that of thiazide diuretics. They are more useful in the treatment of fluid retention, as occurs in congestive heart failure, nephrotic syndrome, or cirrhosis of the liver. In addition, they are used for treatment of hypercalcemia because they lower the plasma calcium concentration by increasing the renal excretion of calcium.

Fluid and electrolyte imbalance is the most common form of clinical toxicity. Hypokalemia can occur with the use of these diuretics, but the total loss of potassium is probably less than that occurs with longer-acting diuretics. Hyperuricemia and hyperglycemia are seen as with thiazide diuretics. Gastrointestinal discomfort, skin rash, paresthesias, and hepatic dysfunction have also been reported. Allergic interstitial nephritis leading to reversible renal failure can occur both with furosemide and thiazides. Transient deafness has been reported with furosemide in large doses. The development of deafness, either transient or permanent, may also be a complication of ethacrynic acid.

Preparations and dosages are indicated in Table 1.

Potassium-sparing diuretics. These include spironolactone (Aldactone) and triamterene (Dyrenium).

Spironolactone is a steroidal compound with a structural formula similar to aldosterone. It is a competitive antagonist of aldosterone and acts on the distal tubule of the nephron. Thus it prevents potassium excretion and sodium absorption at this site. In addition, it increases calcium excretion through a direct effect on tubular transport.

Spironolactone prevents aldosterone-produced hypokalemia. In addition, it potentiates the effect of other diuretics such as thiazides and loop diuretics. This agent has an antihypertensive effect similar to the thiazides and loop diuretics. However, it is probably not as efficacious.

It is absorbed through the gastrointestinal tract and is metabolized in the liver in a manner similar to other steroid hormones.

Spironolactone is indicated in the treatment of hypokalemia and in prevention of hypokalemia induced by other diuretics. It is used to potentiate the antihypertensive and diuretic effects of the thiazides and loop diuretics. It is also used in the medical treatment of patients with primary aldosteronism. A few years ago spironolactone was proposed as a useful agent in the treatment of low-renin hypertension. However, as a sole antihypertensive agent, it has not been a satisfactory drug.

Contraindications include renal insufficiency and hyperkalemia.

Gynecomastia in the male and menstrual irregularity in the female are important side effects. Hyperkalemia can occur but usually only when the patient has renal insufficiency. The reports of spironolactone-induced breast carcinoma have not been substantiated.

Preparations and dosages are indicated in Table 1. Aldactazide is a combination of hydrochlorothiazide (25 mg.) and spironolactone (25 mg.).

Triamterene is chemically related to folic acid but does not have any significant antifolic activity. It has a mild diuretic action in the distal tubule characterized by an increase in the excretion of sodium chloride and water. However, the primary action is inhibition of potassium secretion in the distal nephron. It acts independent of aldosterone and is not its competitive inhibitor.

In addition to potentiating the diuretic action of thiazides and loop diuretics, triamterene causes potassium retention and prevents hypokalemia. It has little antihypertensive effect.

Triamterene is rapidly absorbed from the gastrointestinal tract and is excreted essentially unchanged in the urine. In the plasma, it is about two thirds bound to protein. The urinary excretion is accomplished by both filtration and tubular secretion.

The drug is used primarily to conserve potassium and prevent hypokalemia caused by thiazide and loop diuretics. It is contraindicated in patients with renal insufficiency. Except for occasional reports of gastrointestinal disturbances, photosensitivity, and skin rash, it does not have significant adverse effects.

Preparations and dosages are indicated in Table 1. Dyazide is a combination of hydrochlorothiazide (25 mg.) and triamterene (50 mg.).

Sympathetic inhibitors

Reserpine. A drug frequently added to diuretics is reserpine. By itself, it is a weak hypotensive drug but in combination with a diuretic may be useful.

Reserpine is a purified alkaloid of the Indian snakeroot *Rauwolfia serpentina*. A number of natural and semisynthetic alkaloids other than reserpine are also available.

Reserpine has both central and peripheral sympathoplegic actions. It depletes the stores of catecholamines and prevents their reuptake into the nerve endings (Fig. 8). It acts at the sympathetic nerve endings, in the adrenal medulla, and in some areas of the central nervous system, notably the hypothalamus. It also depletes stores of serotonin, which is stored in mast cells and in platelets.

Reserpine causes a slow fall in blood pressure, frequently associated with bradycardia. Chronic administration is usually associated with a reduced cardiac output. In addition, it produces sedation and tranquilization. The cardiovascular reflexes are maintained, and it seldom causes postural hypotension. In high doses, it can cause extrapyramidal signs as seen in parkinsonism and convulsions.

Reserpine—but not necessarily all its analogues—is well absorbed after oral administration. It requires up to 3 weeks for the full antihypertensive effect to develop. Reserpine is rapidly taken up by the lipid-containing tissues and is uni-

Adrenergic nerve ending   Receptor

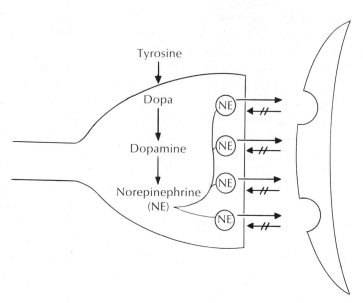

Fig. 8. Adrenergic nerve ending showing the synthesis, storage, release, and reuptake of norepinephrine. Reserpine blocks the reuptake of norepinephrine, and guanethidine depletes the norepinephrine storage granules.

formly distributed in the brain. The drug is metabolized in the liver and excreted in the bile. After discontinuance, the autonomic actions persist for 7 to 10 days. It may be a month before reserpine completely disappears from the blood.

Reserpine is primarily used in the treatment of essential hypertension, always in combination with a diuretic, and often along with a third vasodilator drug. Its use as a tranquilizer has been surpassed by phenothiazines and other agents.

Contraindications include known hypersensitivity, mental depression (especially with suicidal tendencies), active peptic ulcer, ulcerative colitis, allergic sinusitis, and epistaxis. In addition, it is contraindicated for patients receiving electroconvulsive therapy.

Adverse reactions are generally an extension of its pharmacologic actions. The common side effects include nasal stuffiness, depression, increased appetite, weight gain, and excessive gastric secretion with activation of peptic ulcer. Parkinsonism occurs only after large doses. Sexual dysfunction, although not common, can occur in men. Allergic reaction to the *Rauwolfia* alkaloids are relatively rare.

Reserpine (Raurine, Rau-Sed, Reserpoid, Sandril, Serpasil, Serpate, Vio-Serpine) is available in 0.25 and 0.5 mg. capsules; as an elixir, 0.95 mg./ml.; in solution (for injection), 5 mg./2 ml. and 25 or 50 mg./10 ml.; and as tablets, 0.1, 0.25, 0.5, 1, 2 and 5 mg. The usual dose is 0.25 mg./24 hr. orally. The whole root

Rauwolfia serpentina (Raudixin) is supplied in 50 and 100 mg. tablets. The average dose is 200 to 400 mg. daily. It is also marketed in combination with diuretics under various trade names and in combination with hydrochlorothiazide and hydralazine as Ser-Ap-Es, which contains 0.1 mg. reserpine, 25 mg. hydralazine, and 15 mg. hydrochlorothiazide.

Methyldopa (Aldomet). Chemically, methyldopa is L-α-methyl-3,4-dihydroxyphenylalanine, a compound structurally similar to L-dopa.

The mechanism of action of methyldopa as an antihypertensive agent has undergone considerable revision since its discovery as a dopa-decarboxylase inhibitor in 1954. Because methyldopa is itself metabolized to α-methylnorepinephrine, which can be stored in sympathetic nerve endings, it was hypothesized that norepinephrine was displaced in the storage granules by α-methylnorepinephrine, which then acted as a "false transmitter." The current view generally accepted is that the major antihypertensive action of methyldopa is on the central nervous system and is mediated through α-methylnorepinephrine.

Methyldopa causes reduction in blood pressure and heart rate in 1 to 2 hours after administration. The maximum effect occurs in 4 to 6 hours and persists for as long as 24 hours after a single oral dose. The fall in blood pressure is greater in hypertensive than in normotensive subjects. It is reported to reduce cardiac output and peripheral resistance. It also decreases plasma renin activity but tends to cause sodium and water retention. Since the blood pressure is lower in the upright than the supine position, orthostatic hypotension may occur but is not common. Renal blood flow and glomerular filtration rate may be increased.

It produces mild sedation and in large doses can cause hypothermia. After oral administration, approximately 50% of the dose is absorbed rapidly. Most of the drug is excreted unchanged. The rest is excreted as α-methyldopamine and its metabolites. Its presence in the urine can cause false positive tests for pheochromocytoma.

Methyldopa is used in treatment of hypertension when the effect of a thiazide diuretic is not adequate. If the two drugs are insufficient in controlling hypertension adequately, a vasodilator is usually added.

It is contraindicated in the presence of active hepatic disease such as acute hepatitis, cirrhosis of the liver, and when there is a past history of liver disorder.

Mild sedation is not uncommon. However, persistent lassitude and drowsiness may be particularly disturbing to some patients. Postural hypotension with dizziness may develop. Almost 20% of patients may develop a positive Coombs' test, but frank hemolytic anemia is uncommon. A hypersensitivity reaction involving the liver can occur within weeks of starting methyldopa and is usually reversible. Rare adverse reactions include drug fever, granulocytopenia, and thrombocytopenia.

Methyldopa (Aldomet) is available for oral administration in tablets containing 125, 250, and 500 mg. It is also available in 5 ml. vials (50 mg./ml.) for intravenous use. Many patients respond to a single dose of 250 mg. daily when added to a diuretic. The dose can be increased up to 2 gm./24 hr. given in two to four divided doses. It is also available in combination with hydrochlorothiazide as Aldoril-15 (methyldopa, 250 mg. and hydrochlorothiazide, 15 mg.) and Aldoril-25 (methyldopa, 250 mg., and hydrochlorothiazide, 25 mg.). Combination with chlorothiazide is named Aldoclor. It is available as Aldoclor-150 (methyldopa, 250 mg., and chlorothiazide, 150 mg.), and Aldoclor-250 (methyldopa, 250 mg., and chlorothiazide, 250 mg.).

Clonidine (Catapres). Clonidine is an imidazoline derivative closely related chemically to tolazoline, a peripheral vasodilator.

It causes a decrease in sympathetic outflow from the brain by inhibition of the bulbar sympathetic vasoconstrictor centers. It also stimulates peripheral adrenergic receptors, producing transient vasoconstriction.

The blood pressure declines within 30 to 60 minutes after an oral dose, the maximum decrease occurring within 2 to 4 hours. The antihypertensive effect lasts approximately 6 to 8 hours. The orthostatic effects are mild and infrequent, and clonidine does not alter normal hemodynamic responses to exercise. Slowing of the pulse rate has been observed in most patients given clonidine. Studies have demonstrated reductions in plasma renin activity and excretion of aldosterone and catecholamines after administration of clonidine.

The drug is rapidly absorbed after oral administration. Approximately 32% is excreted unchanged in the urine. The remainder is metabolized and also excreted in the urine.

Clonidine is used as an alternative to reserpine or methyldopa in the treatment of hypertension and is always given in combination with a diuretic. It is useful in the control of mild to moderate hypertension. This drug has been found effective in reducing the number of attacks of migraine and vascular instability associated with menopause. However, these two uses are still investigational.

There are no specific contraindications to the use of clonidine. However, it should be avoided during pregnancy and in children, since the safety of the drug has not been established in these situations.

Dry mouth, drowsiness, and sedation are the most common side effects. Constipation, dizziness, headaches, and fatigue have also been reported. On abrupt cessation of therapy, acute hypertensive crisis and encephalopathy have been reported. When discontinuing clonidine, it should be reduced over a period of 2 to 4 days.

Clonidine (Catapres) is marketed in 0.1 and 0.2 mg. tablets. The initial dose is 0.1 mg. twice daily. Further increments of 0.1 or 0.2 mg./24 hr. are made until the desired antihypertensive response is achieved. The maximum daily dose is 2 mg. daily. Combipress 0.1 and Combipress 0.2 are combinations of clonidine 0.1 and 0.2 mg., respectively, with 15 mg. chlorthalidone (Hygroton) in each tablet.

Trimethaphan (Arfonad). Trimethaphan is a ganglionic blocking agent presently used for treatment of hypertension. Tetraethylammonium (TEA) and hexamethonium are other ganglionic blocking drugs of historical significance. Mecamylamine (Inversine) and pentolinium (Ansolysen) are also ganglion blockers that are still available but used rarely in the treatment of hypertension.

Trimethaphan is a thiophanium compound. It blocks both the sympathetic and parasympathetic ganglia. It acts by occupying receptor sites on the ganglion cells and by stabilizing the postsynaptic membrane against the action of acetylcholine liberated from the presynaptic nerve endings. In addition to ganglion blocking, trimethaphan also exerts a direct peripheral vasodilator effect and liberates histamine.

It produces both arteriolar and venous dilation, producing a fall in blood pressure. The venous dilation with peripheral pooling of blood results in a decrease in cardiac output. The pulse rate increases. The gastrointestinal motility is decreased, causing constipation sometimes to the point of ileus.

Trimethaphan is available only for intravenous use. After its introduction into the circulation, it is confined primarily to the extracellular space. Penetration of the blood-brain barrier is limited. Most of the drug is excreted unchanged by the kidney.

It is indicated for the short-term (acute) control of blood pressure in hypertensive emergencies such as acute dissecting aneurysm of the aorta. It is also used for production of controlled hypotension during surgery and in the emergency treatment of pulmonary edema in patients with acute left ventricular failure associated with systemic hypertension. Trimethaphan is contraindicated in cases in which hypotension may subject the patient to undue risks. Examples of such conditions include uncorrected anemia, hypovolemia, shock, asphyxia, or uncorrected respiratory insufficiency.

Because of parasympathetic blockade, trimethaphan produces urinary retention, dry mouth, loss of ocular accommodation, pupillary dilation, and impotence. Chest pain may be precipitated in patients with angina pectoris if the hypotension is excessive. Sometimes syncope may occur without warning.

Trimethaphan must always be diluted and administered by intravenous infusion. Solutions should be freshly prepared and unused portions discarded. Trimethaphan camsylate (Arfonad) is available in 10 ml. ampules containing 50 mg./ml. For administration, one ampule (500 mg.) should be diluted in 500 ml. of 5% dextrose. The rate of administration must be adjusted to the requirements of each patient. It is started at an average rate of 60 drops (3 to 4 mg.) per minute. Frequent blood pressure determinations are essential to maintain proper control. The patient is best treated with an intraarterial line in place and cardiac monitor attached.

Guanethidine (Ismelin). Guanethidine, bretylium, bethanidine, and debrisoquin are adrenergic neuron blocking agents. They are also called "postganglionic blocking agents." Of these, only guanethidine is available for clinical use in the United States.

Guanethidine has a guanidine group, a strongly basic moiety. It is taken up slowly by the sympathetic nerve endings just as norepinephrine is taken up and replaces norepinephrine in cytoplasm and granules of the nerve. After 3 to 5 days, sympathetic nerves contain and release less norepinephrine. Thus guanethidine interferes with chemical mediation at the postganglionic adrenergic nerve endings (Fig. 8). In addition, it has considerable local anesthetic activity. The norepinephrine depletion persists for several days after the drug has been discontinued. It has little effect on the catecholamine content of the adrenal medulla and penetrates the central nervous system poorly. Tricyclic antidepressants such as amitriptyline (Elavil) displace guanethidine from the nerve endings, thus reversing its effect. Guanethidine can also be released by reserpine, amphetamine, and tyramine, the second two drugs decreasing its antihypertensive response.

Guanethidine causes a fall in blood pressure, which is most intense in the upright posture. The pulse rate is slowed, and an increase in gastrointestinal motility is seen. Diarrhea is common. Ejaculation may be delayed or prevented, but erection is usually not a problem.

It is well absorbed after oral administration, but the pharmacologic effect develops slowly. It is metabolized in the liver, and the parent drug and metabolites are excreted in the urine. A limited degree of tolerance develops during prolonged treatment with guanethidine, but simultaneous administration of a diuretic prevents this.

Guanethidine is used in the treatment of severe hypertension, usually after a diuretic and one of the other antihypertensives have been tried. The diuretic is continued and the other antihypertensive replaced by guanethidine. Its use is under investigation in the treatment of hyperthyroidism.

It is contraindicated if pheochromocytoma is suspected, since catecholamine released from the nerve endings by guanethidine may cause a hypertensive crisis. It is also contraindicated in congestive heart failure.

Dizziness and fainting are undesirable effects, resulting from postural hypotension. Diarrhea may be severe at times and necessitate use of atropine analogues or discontinuance of guanethidine. Inhibition of ejaculation, fluid retention, urinary incontinence, blurred vision, and nasal congestion are some other side effects.

Guanethidine (Ismelin) is available in 10 and 25 mg. tablets for oral administration. The usual daily dose is 25 to 50 mg., but it varies widely. A single daily dose is usually satisfactory. As an outpatient the starting dose is generally 10 mg. daily, which is increased at intervals of about a week until the desired effects are obtained. A higher initial dose may be administered to inpatients and increased more rapidly.

Phentolamine (Regitine) and phenoxybenzamine (Dibenzyline). These two drugs are α-adrenergic receptor blocking agents. Ahlquist proposed the terms "alpha (α) and beta (β) receptors" for adrenoceptive sites on smooth muscles where catecholamines produce excitation and inhibition. In most blood vessels, stimulation of α receptors produces vasoconstriction and that of β receptors, vasodilation. In the gut, stimulation of both α and β receptors produce relaxation. Sympathetic stimulation of the heart increases its rate (chronotropic effect) and force of contraction (inotropic effect), both being mediated by β adrenergic receptors. Isoproterenol (Isuprel) is the most potent β stimulating agent. Epinephrine and norepinephrine possess both α and β stimulatory properties. However, norepinephrine is primarily an α stimulator and has much less β stimulating actions than epinephrine.

Phentolamine is an imidazoline derivative similar to tolazoline and other vasodepressor compounds. It produces a moderately effective competitive α adrenergic blockage that is relatively transient. Response to serotonin is also inhibited. Gastric secretion of acid and pepsin is also stimulated. It decreases peripheral resistance and increases venous capacity, causing a fall in blood pressure. The dilation is predominately due to a direct action on vascular smooth muscle and α blockade occurs at a higher dose. In patients with pheochromocytoma, administration of phentolamine produces a precipitous fall in blood pressure and may even cause the patient to go into shock.

Only 10% of an injected dose of phentolamine can be recovered in the urine in active form. It is only 20% as active after oral as after parenteral administration. Little is known about the fate of the drug in the body.

Phentolamine is primarily used to prevent or control hypertension in a patient with pheochromocytoma preoperatively, intraoperatively, and when the tumor is inoperable. It is also used as a blocking agent in pharmacologic diagnosis of pheochromocytoma. With the advent of biochemical tests for the diagnosis of pheochromocytoma, the pharmacologic tests are now seldom necessary. Prevention and treatment of dermal necrosis and sloughing from extravasation following intravenous administration of norepinephrine are other indications for the use of phentolamine.

Contraindications include coronary artery disease and hypersensitivity to phentolamine or related compounds. Acute and prolonged hypotensive episodes, cardiac arrhythmias, and tachycardia are the most frequent side effects after parenteral administration.

Phentolamine (Regitine) is marketed for parenteral use in sterile ampules containing 5 mg. It is also available for oral use in tablets containing 50 mg.

Phenoxybenzamine is a haloalkylamine, chemically related to nitrogen mustard. It is a long-acting, α-adrenergic receptor blocking agent that can produce and maintain chemical sympathectomy.

It increases blood flow to the skin, mucosa, and abdominal viscera and lowers both supine and upright blood pressures. This agent has no effect on the parasympathetic system.

Approximately 20% to 30% of orally administered phenoxybenzamine is absorbed in the active form. It is lipid soluble at body pH and is bound to tissues in a stable fashion. Most of the drug is excreted within 24 hours of administration. Phenoxybenzamine is used to control episodes of hypertension and sweating in patients with pheochromocytoma. It is generally used in combination with a β blocking agent in this situation. It may also be useful in vasospastic peripheral vascular disorders such as Raynaud's syndrome, acrocyanosis, and frostbite.

Phenoxybenzamine is contraindicated when a fall in blood pressure may be undesirable.

Side effects are due to extension of the adrenergic blockade and vary according to its intensity. Nasal congestion, postural hypotension, tachycardia, and inhibition of ejaculation may occur.

Phenoxybenzamine (Dibenzyline) is available for oral use in 10 mg. capsules. It is available for intravenous use for investigational purposes. The oral dose varies between 20 and 200 mg./24 hr. and must be attained by small increments.

Propranolol (Inderal). The first drug shown to produce a selective blockade of β-adrenergic receptors was dichloroisoproterenol (DCI). Propranolol is currently the only β-adrenergic blocking agent on the market in the United States and Canada, although others are available elsewhere. They differ in potency and β receptor selectivity. The β-adrenergic receptors of various tissues can be differentiated pharmacologically as β_1 (e.g., in the heart) and β_2 (e.g., in most smooth muscles).

Propranolol, like most of the other β-adrenergic blocking agents, is a derivative of the β receptor stimulator, isoproterenol. The β-adrenergic receptor–blocking drugs compete specifically with β-adrenergic receptor–stimulating agents for available receptor sites. The mechanism of the antihypertensive effects of propranolol has not been established. Among the factors that may be involved are (1) decreased cardiac output, (2) inhibition of renin released by the kidneys, and (3) diminution of tonic sympathetic nerve outflow from vasomotor centers in the brain. In dosages greater than required for β blockade, propranolol also exerts a quinidine-like or anesthetic-like membrane action that affects the cardiac action potential and depresses cardiac function. This makes propranolol a useful antiarrhythmic drug. It blocks the effects of catecholamines on carbohydrate and fat metabolism mediated through β-adrenergic receptors and changes adenyl-cyclase activity.

Propranolol decreases heart rate, cardiac output, and blood pressure. Recent studies suggest that in the absence of sodium restriction, plasma volume may increase. It reduces the oxygen requirement of the heart at any given level of effort, which makes it a useful drug in the treatment of angina. Even in normal subjects the administration of propranolol causes bronchiolar constriction. Patients with asthma or other obstructive pulmonary diseases are especially susceptible to this effect.

Propranolol is indicated as a second drug in the treatment of hypertension if the patient has not responded to diuretic therapy alone. Laragh[2] suggests that propranolol be used as a drug of first choice in the treatment of essential hypertension because of its low toxicity and better patient tolerance. However, most other experts believe that in view of the large experience accumulated with the use of diuretics, these should be the drug of first choice and propranolol used as a second step drug. Investigations need to be conducted using propranolol as the first step drug and and comparisons made with diuretic therapy. Propranolol is also useful in the treatment of certain arrhythmias, symptoms of thyrotoxicosis, hypertrophic aortic stenosis, pheochromocytoma, and angina.

Contraindications to the use of propranolol are congestive heart failure, bronchial asthma, brittle diabetes, and bradycardia.

Side effects may be common early in the treatment but tend to disappear or are greatly reduced with continued administration of the drug. They include dizziness, tiredness, depression, increased dreaming, gastrointestinal disturbances, parasthesias, and asthmatic wheezing. Impotence has also been reported with the use of propranolol.

Propranolol is available in tablets containing 10, 40, and 80 mg. for oral administration and in 1 ml. ampules containing 1 mg. for intravenous use. The dose range of propranolol is different for each indication. For treatment of hypertension, the initial dose is 80 mg./24 hr. in two divided doses. The dose may be gradually increased until optimum blood pressure response is achieved. Although higher doses have been administered, the usual dose range is 40 to 480 mg./24 hr.

Intravenous propranolol is useful in control of hypertension in patients with pheochromocytoma during surgery and in the treatment of arrhythmias.

Vasodilators

Hydralazine (Apresoline). Hydralazine is a phthalazine derivative. Minoxidil and guancydine are two other distant congeners of hydralazine with similar hemodynamic effects and considerable antihypertensive activity but are not yet available for clinical use in the United States.

The major action of hydralazine is direct relaxation of the vascular smooth muscle, the effect on arteries being greater than on veins. The consequent fall in blood pressure produces a reflex cardiac stimulation, causing tachycardia. The primary effect of hydralazine is to decrease peripheral resistance, causing a fall in blood pressure. The reflex tachycardia leads to increased cardiac output. Hydralazine is well absorbed from the gastrointestinal tract. The blood levels are maximal in 3 to 4 hours. This agent has a high affinity for the walls of muscular arteries. It is metabolized in the liver by conjugation with glucuronic acid and by N-acetylation. Only a small fraction is excreted unchanged.

The primary indication for use of hydralazine is essential hypertension when diuretics and a sympathetic inhibitor drug are insufficient in controlling blood pressure.

It is also recommended in the treatment of congestive heart failure when diuretic and digitalis therapy are insufficient. By vasodilation, it reduces the peripheral resistance (afterload, impedence) and thus allows peripheral pooling of the blood.

Hypersensitivity to hydralazine is a contraindication to its use. Coronary artery disease and angina are relative contraindications to its use because the reflex tachycardia may cause overt myocardial infarction. For the same reason it is also contraindicated in mitral valvular rheumatic heart disease. Headache, palpitations, tachycardia, and angina pectoris are relatively common side effects. Less frequent side effects include nasal congestion, lupuslike syndrome, and blood dyscrasias.

Hydralazine (Apresoline) is available in 10, 25, 50, and 100 mg. tablets for oral administration and in 1 ml. ampules containing 20 mg. of the drug for parenteral use. The drug is started with 10 to 20 mg. daily in two divided doses and increased gradually up to 100 to 200 mg./24 hr. until the desired effect is obtained or unacceptable side effects develop.

Apresazide is a combination of hydralazine and hydrochlorothiazide available as 25-25, 50-50, and 100-50 capsules containing that many milligrams of hydralazine and hydrochlorothiazide, respectively.

Prazosin (Minipress). Prazosin is a quinazoline derivative and is the first of a new chemical class of antihypertensives.

This drug acts as a direct smooth muscle relaxant. Blood pressure depression is believed to be due to direct relaxation of peripheral arterioles and is associated with decreased total peripheral resistance. It probably acts by increasing cyclic adenosine monophosphate (AMP) levels in arteriolar smooth muscle cells. Prazosin may also have a sympatholytic effect on the heart. Blood pressure is lowered more in the standing than the supine position. The fall in blood pressure is usually not accompanied by a clinically significant change in cardiac output, heart rate, renal blood flow, and glomerular filtration rate. It does not increase plasma renin activity. The effect is more pronounced on the diastolic blood pressure.

Following oral administration, plasma concentrations reach a peak level at 3 hours with a plasma half-life of 2 to 3 hours. The drug is highly bound to plasma protein. It is extensively metabolized in the liver by demethylation and conjugation and excreted mainly in the bile. Prazosin is indicated in treatment of mild to moderate hypertension in conjunction with a diuretic. When combined with methyldopa and a diuretic, it is useful in control of severe hypertension. It is contraindicated in patients who have experienced syncopal episodes for any reason.

Prazosin has been reported to cause syncope (with sudden loss of consciousness) after the first dose in rare instances. Syncopal episodes are not always associated with postural hypotension. Certain patients may feel dizzy and light-headed because of postural hypotension. Drowsiness, lack of energy, weakness, palpitations, and nausea are some other effects seen with prazosin.

Prazosin (Minipress) is available in 1, 2, and 5 mg. capsules. The initial recommended dose is 1 mg. three times a day. The first dose preferably should be given at bedtime to avoid syncopal episodes. The dose should be adjusted to the patient's blood pressure response. Generally, 20 mg./24 hr. is the maximum dose.

Sodium nitroprusside (Nipride). This is a powerful antihypertensive agent that was used sporadically for almost forty years. It is now commercially available for treatment of hypertensive emergencies.

Sodium nitroprusside is a nitrite compound containing sodium nitroprusside dihydrate. It is a potent and rapid-acting vasodilator. The effect of this agent is almost immediate and ends when the intravenous infusion is stopped. It causes a rapid fall in arterial and central venous pressures and a moderate increase in heart rate. Cardiac output is slightly increased. Vascular dilation is not as pronounced in the renal vascular bed. It has no effect on smooth muscle other than that of blood vessels.

After intravenous administration, sodium nitroprusside is rapidly converted into thiocyanate and the effect terminated.

It is used for short-term, rapid reduction in blood pressure in treatment of hypertensive emergencies. This agent is also useful for producing hypotension in minimizing bleeding during surgery. It has also been shown to improve left ventricular function after acute myocardial infarction. The use of this drug in chronic refractory heart failure has been encouraging.

It is contraindicated where facilities for continuous monitoring of the blood pressure do not exist, since the fall in arterial blood pressure is dose dependent and does not reach a "floor."

The acute toxicity of nitroprusside is secondary to excessive vasodilation and hypotension. With prolonged therapy (2 to 3 weeks), cyanide and thiocyanate may accumulate. Cyanide toxicity is extremely uncommon, but temporary hypothyroidism from the effect of thiocyanate can occur.

Sodium nitroprusside (Nipride) is a reddish brown, water-soluble powder marketed in 5 ml. amber-colored vials, each containing 50 mg. of the drug. Only a fresh solution (less than 4 hours old) should be used. Solution is made first by adding 2 to 3 ml. dextrose solution in water to the vial and then transferring the contents to an infusion bottle containing 500 ml. of the same diluent. Because the compound decomposes in light, the bottle should be covered with an opaque wrapping, usually an aluminum foil. It should be administered only by slow intravenous infusion using a microdrip regulator to ensure precise flow rate. Meticulous care should be taken to prevent extravasation. The average adult dose is 200 μg./min. but the range of dosage is broad. The objective is to reduce the blood pressure to an acceptable level. Continuous monitoring of the patient, blood pressure, and flow rate is absolutely essential.

Diazoxide (Hyperstat). Diazoxide is chemically related to the thiazide diuretics, although it is not a diuretic. It directly dilates arterioles and has little effect on the veins. A rapid intravenous injection produces a marked antihypertensive effect, which usually persists for 4 to 12 hours. It is accompanied by a considerable increase in cardiac output and tachycardia. Generally, the blood pressure does not fall below the normal range, and postural hypotension usually does not develop. It causes marked retention of sodium and water, the opposite

Table 2. Commonly used antihypertensives

Generic name	Trade name	Size of tablets (mg.)	Usual dose range (mg./24 hr.)	Contraindications
Sympathetic inhibitors				
Reserpine and analogues	Many	0.1, 0.25, 0.5, 1, 2, and 5	0.1-2	Mental depression, peptic ulcer, obesity, epistaxis, sinusitis
Methyldopa	Aldomet	125, 250, and 500	250-2000	Liver disease, hemolytic anemia
Clonidine	Catapres	0.1 and 0.2	0.1-2	None
Trimethaphan	Arfonad	IV infusion only 500 mg./10 ml. ampule	500 mg. in 500 ml. of 5% dextrose in water Start 3-4 mg./min., increase to titrate BP	Uncorrected anemia, hypovolemia, asphyxia, uncorrected respiratory insufficiency, glaucoma
Guanethidine	Ismelin	10 and 25	10-100	Sexual dysfunction, pheochromocytoma, congestive heart failure
Propranolol	Inderal	10, 40, and 80	40-480	Congestive heart failure, asthma, brittle diabetes, bradycardia
Vasodilators				
Hydralazine	Apresoline	10, 25, 50, and 100	20-200	Angina, mitral valve disease, SLE, syncopal episodes
Prazosin	Minipress	1, 2, and 5	3-20	Syncope
Sodium nitroprusside	Nipride	IV infusion only 50 mg./5 ml. ampule	50 mg. in 500 ml. of 5% dextrose in water Start 200 μg./min., increase to titrate BP	Absence of facilities for continuous BP monitoring
Diazoxide	Hyperstat	IV push only 300 mg./20 ml. ampule	300-600 mg. rapid IV push	Angina, uncontrolled diabetes, heart failure

of thiazide diuretics. These effects can, however, be antagonized by a diuretic. In common with thiazides, it inhibits tubular excretion of uric acid and produces glucose intolerance.

Intravenous diazoxide binds rapidly to plasma proteins. The plasma half-life is 24 to 36 hours; however, the antihypertensive effect lasts less than 12 hours. Intravenous diazoxide is used for the treatment of accelerated and malignant hypertension in hospitalized patients when prompt and urgent decrease of diastolic blood pressure is required.

It should not be used in patients hypersensitive to thiazides and sulfonamides.

The major side effects are salt and water retention, hyperglycemia, and hyperuricemia. Chronic administration has been reported to cause hypertrichosis (excessive hairiness).

Diazoxide (Hyperstat I.V.) is available for intravenous use in 20 ml. ampules containing 300 mg. of the drug. It is alkaline, and meticulous care must be taken to avoid extravasation. The usual dose is 300 to 600 mg. injected intravenously rapidly.

Tablet size, usual dose, and contraindications of the commonly used antihypertensives are summarized in Table 2.

SUMMARY

The antihypertensive drugs play a major role in the treatment of hypertension. Medications used in the treatment of hypertension include diuretics, sympathetic inhibitors, and vasodilators. Thiazides are the most commonly used diuretics. They act by decreasing blood volume and slight vasodilation. Furosemide and ethacrynic acid produce marked diuresis and are effective antihypertensives. Spironolactone is an antialdosterone compound that is usually used in combination with a thiazide diuretic to prevent excessive potassium loss. Triamterene is also a potassium-conserving agent. The long-acting diuretics offer the advantage of less frequent dosage.

The sympathetic inhibitors include reserpine, methyldopa, clonidine, guanethidine, and the β blocker propranolol. These are efficacious antihypertensive agents used in combination with a diuretic for treatment of moderate to moderately severe hypertension. The ganglion blocker trimethaphan is used as an intravenous infusion in reducing blood pressure in patients with dissecting aneurysm of aorta. The α blockers phentolamine and phenoxybenazamine along with propranolol are employed in the medical treatment of pheochromocytoma.

The vasodilators hydralazine and prazosin are utilized in the treatment of severe hypertension. They are usually used in combination with a diuretic and a sympathetic inhibitor. Sodium nitroprusside is an effective hypotensive agent and is always used in the form of a slow intravenous infusion with close monitoring of blood pressure. Diazoxide is chemically similar to thiazides but is not a diuretic. It is a vasodilator used in the management of hypertensive emergencies.

SUGGESTED READINGS

1. Goodman, L. S., and Gilman, A.: The pharmacological basis of therapeutics, ed. 5, New York, 1975, Macmillan Publishing Co., Inc.
2. Larargh, J. H.: Modern system for treating high blood pressure based on renin profiling and vaso-constriction-volume analysis: a primary role for beta blocking drugs such as propranolol, Am. J. Med. **61:**797-810, 1976.
3. Physician's desk reference, ed. 32, Oradell, N.J., 1978, Medical Economics Co.

CHAPTER 4

Evaluation of the hypertensive patient

Before treatment of a hypertensive patient can be undertaken, it is necessary that a proper evaluation of the disease be conducted. The evaluation process consists of a detailed history, an appropriate physical examination, and certain laboratory tests. The history is probably the most important of these.

PURPOSE OF EVALUATION

The purpose of evaluation is to seek answers to the following questions:
1. *Does the patient have hypertension?* The patient may have been referred after one or two readings of his blood pressure. If a patient is found to have an elevated reading on one occasion, there is a 70% chance that he will have high blood pressure on subsequent measurements. If the blood pressure is elevated on two occasions, there is a 90% chance that it will be high on subsequent measurements. Generally, the blood pressure is higher in a physician's office than it is in a screening setting. If an individual is found to have normal blood pressure in the physician's office but has elevated readings during the screening, he may have labile hypertension and may need follow-up with or without pharmacologic therapy. If blood pressure readings are repeatedly normal in a physician's office, it is possible that the high readings during the screening were erroneous.

2. *Is it likely that the patient has secondary hypertension requiring further investigations?* Depending on the patient population, between 3% and 5% of patients with hypertension may have a primary disorder such as renal, endocrine, or vascular disease causing hypertension. In certain instances, surgical treatment of the primary disorder may cure hypertension or make it easier to control with medical therapy. By means of the evaluation process, it should be possible to suspect the presence of one of these disorders and then undertake certain other laboratory and radiologic investigations to prove the diagnosis.

3. *What is the extent of target organ damage?* Although patients may be unaware of their hypertension, they may have had the condition for several months or years prior to the diagnosis. Thus hypertension and atherosclerosis may have already caused cardiac, cerebrovascular, and renal damage. Although the treatment of hypertension is helpful in preventing further damage, it is unlikely to reverse what has already occurred. The future prognosis in terms of morbidity and mortality depends on the extent of end organ damage already present.

4. *What other "risk factors" are present?* The primary reason for control of hypertension is to prevent its complications. As pointed out previously, atherosclerosis is the major complication of hypertension, which leads to coronary artery disease, cerebrovascular disease, and renal damage. Although hypertension is the major risk factor leading to atherosclerosis, other contributing causes include high cholesterol level, diabetes mellitus, family history of atherosclerosis, obesity, and others mentioned in Chapter 1. The purpose of the evaluation of hypertensive patients is to detect these risk factors so that appropriate steps can be taken to correct them simultaneous with hypertension control.

5. *Are there conditions present that would contraindicate certain antihypertensive drugs?* Diuretics, the most commonly used antihypertensive agents, may produce hyperuricemia, hyperglycemia, hypokalemia, and hyperlipidemia. Although the presence of these conditions are not considered contraindications to diuretic therapy, patients who already have one or more of these conditions require appropriate precautions when prescribing treatment. Asthma, severe allergic sinusitis, brittle diabetes, and bradycardia are contraindications to propranolol therapy. Patients with liver disease should not be treated with methyldopa, which can produce further liver damage. An adequate evaluation would indicate the presence of these conditions.

6. *What is the patient's life-style?* This applies particularly to diet, smoking, alcohol intake, use of oral contraceptive pills, sleep, and exercise patterns.

7. *What is the patient's level of understanding and attitude toward the disease?* This knowledge would assist the health care professional in individualizing planning and treatment and in making more reliable predictions for compliance.

The history and physical examination form used in our hypertension clinic is shown in the boxed material on pp. 50 to 52. With slight modifications the format can be applied in almost any situation in which hypertension is evaluated and treated.

HISTORY

After the patient is identified, the first question asked relates to the duration of hypertension and previous treatment. Commonly, patients will recall being informed of high blood pressure in the past at armed forces, insurance, or pre-employment physicals. At that time they may have been asked to rest awhile for a second blood pressure reading. Although informed of the elevated reading and possibly advised to consult a physician, patients often do not obtain medical evaluation and treatment. In many instances, even after treatment is initiated, they are not made aware that routine visits to monitor progression and prescription renewal are necessary. Their perception may be that after the medication is finished, the high blood pressure is "cured" and will remain so.

Prolonged duration of hypertension would strongly indicate target organ damage. On the other hand, if the patient had a normal blood pressure 6 months ago but now it is severely elevated, the hypertension is probably secondary in nature.

Although most patients with mild to moderate hypertension are asymptomatic and are surprised to find that their blood pressure is elevated, it is not unusual for the severely hypertensive to be symptomatic. *Headache,* when present, is typically located in the occipital region and is worse on rising in the morning. Many patients may give a history of awakening during the night with severe occipital headache, which improves on standing and walking after a few minutes. In the supine posture, the cerebrospinal fluid (CSF) pressure increases, causing a headache. On resuming the upright posture, the CSF pressure drops, and the headache disappears. The tension headache, on the other hand, is usually frontal and progresses during the day.

Epistaxis (nosebleed) is not a common manifestation of hypertension. If the blood pressure is recorded at the onset of epistaxis, it is almost always elevated when the epistaxis is secondary to hypertension. It may be a safety mechanism on the body's part to relieve the severe hypertension and thus helps prevent apoplexy (cerebral hemorrhage). Epistaxis is more common in black men than white men, especially under the age of 50 years.

Cardiovascular symptoms such as angina, dyspnea, and ankle edema are late symptoms seen only when coronary artery disease has occurred, causing the heart to fail. Intermittent claudication (leg pain when walking) is indicative of arteriosclerosis of lower extremity arteries. During exercise, the oxygen demand by the muscles increases but because of compromised circulation, ischemia of skeletal muscles occurs and the patient experiences leg pain. This pain almost always disappears on resting. As the disease progresses, the patient is able to walk less and less distance without experiencing pain.

HISTORY

Name and address: _____ Number: _____

_____

Duration of hypertension and previous treatment: _____

Current symptoms

Headaches: Yes/No _____

Epistaxis: Yes/No _____

Cardiovascular

   Chest pain with exertion: Yes/No _____

   Dyspnea: Yes/No _____

   Ankle edema: Yes/No _____

   Leg pain upon walking: Yes/No _____

Cerebrovascular

   Dizziness: Yes/No _____

   Blackouts: Yes/No _____

   Numbness: Yes/No _____

   Blurring of vision despite glasses: Yes/No _____

Renal

   Nocturia: Yes/No _____

   Dysuria: Yes/No _____

   Urine infection (past or present):   Yes/No _____

   Past history of kidney disease: Yes/No _____

Pheo symptoms (episodes of palpitation, perspiration, and pallor):

   Yes/No _____

Aldo symptoms (fatigue, nocturia, increased thirst):   Yes/No _____

Other symptoms: _____

_____

_____

Date and reason for last visit to a physician: _____

Significant past illnesses and operations: _____

_____

_____

HISTORY—cont'd

Family history

	A/D	Age	HBP	Heart disease	Diabetes	Stroke	Kidney disease
Father:							
Mother:							
Siblings:							
Children:							

Other relatives (specify who): _____

Who do you live with now? _____

Personal history

Diet: Who cooks? _____

Food preferences: (please circle)   High-salt diet   Fried foods   Cheese
   Eggs   Fruits   Green vegetables   Licorice   Others _____

Smoking: _____

Alcohol: _____

Drug abuse: _____

Exercise: _____

Sleep: _____

Employment and source of income: _____

Education: Ability to read and write: _____

Pregnancies: _____

LMP: _____

Birth control pills: _____

Medications (including over-the-counter preparations): _____

Allergies (including asthma and sinus condition): _____

Other salient history: _____

Signature _____ R.N.
Date _____

Continued.

PHYSICAL EXAM

General appearance: _____

Weight (without shoes and coat): _____ Height: _____

Pulse: _____ Peripheral pulses: Radial: _____
Carotids: _____
Femorals: _____

	Sitting	Standing		
BP R. arm:	_____	_____	Leg BP	R. _____
BP L. arm:	_____	_____	(if taken):	L. _____

Fundi: _____

Neck: _____
Heart:
Size: _____

Rhythm: _____

Sounds: _____

Murmur: _____

Chest: _____

Abdomen and back: _____

Organomegaly: _____

Tenderness: _____

Bruit: _____

Extremities (edema): _____

Skin and hair distribution: _____

Neurologic exam and DTRs: _____

Other significant findings: _____

Clinical impression: _____

Signature _____
Date _____

Cerebrovascular symptoms in the form of dizziness, blackouts, numbness or weakness on one side, and blurring of vision may occur from the effects of hypertension alone or may be indicative of atherosclerosis in the cerebrovascular system. Episodes of numbness and/or weakness on one side of the body usually suggests transient ischemic attack (TIA), which is often a forerunner to a stroke.

The patient with a *pheochromocytoma,* or a tumor of the adrenal medulla, experiences episodic severe headache, palpitation, perspiration, and pallor resulting from excessive secretion of the catecholamines.

Symptoms of *primary aldosteronism* include muscle fatigue because of potassium loss and increased thirst, probably due to sodium retention.

The patient is asked to report and describe other symptoms that he may have experienced in addition to those already mentioned.

The *date and reason for the patient's last visit* to a physician should be recorded along with a blood pressure reading, if known. It is not unusual for a patient to have hypertension and not be informed by the physician. The physician may believe that the blood pressure is elevated because of the stress of a visit to the physician's office, an injury, pain, or other presenting complaint. Another common practice is for the physician to inform the patient of elevated blood pressure, asking him to return for a second reading, but since the patient feels asymptomatic, he fails to return.

Significant past illnesses and operations are also recorded. The patient may have been hospitalized and thoroughly evaluated for hypertension already. He may have been told that there is no cause for his high blood pressure, which the patient interprets as meaning that there is nothing wrong. Although such patients have essential hypertension and should be on lifelong therapy, treatment is not initiated and the patient is not followed up.

The *family history* is important information that must be recorded. The patient should be questioned about the health of his first-degree relatives (father, mother, siblings, children), particularly with regard to hypertension, heart disease, diabetes, stroke, and kidney disease. If any are ill or dead, the age and medical condition should be recorded.

Rather than asking the marital status of a patient, we find it more informative to ask *who the patient is living with at the present time.* "Significant others" in the patient's life can be effectively utilized to promote compliance.

The *personal history* is an extremely important part of the evaluation. The *dietary history* starts with the question, "Who cooks the food?" If the patient lives alone and/or often frequents restaurants that are of the "fast-food" type, he may have little control over how the food is cooked. In that case, he will have to learn to order foods that are less salty. If excessive amounts of salt are added during cooking, it may be necessary to obtain the help of the person who does the cooking to use less salt. If the patient is fond of fried foods, he may be consuming excessive cholesterol. Regular intake of green vegetables and fruits assures adequate potassium intake.

Information about *smoking habits and the type of cigarette smoked* is important to record. The risk of occasional cigarette, pipe, or cigar smoking is minimal. However, the cardiovascular damage produced by smoking one or more packs a day is great.

The patient's *alcohol consumption* is a necessary part of the history. This question needs to be asked gently and cautiously. Most patients underestimate the amount of alcohol consumed and do not readily volunteer the information often.

A patient's history of *drug abuse* is extremely important, since drugs like amphetamines produce vasoconstriction and elevate blood pressure. Furthermore, intravenous amphetamine is reported to cause vasculitis in the kidneys and leads to persistent hypertension.

The *pattern of daily exercise* should be recorded. As explained in Chapter 6, exercise has a role in the management of hypertension. It is important to inquire about the patient's *sleeping habits,* since blood pressure falls during sleep and insomnia may make blood pressure control sometimes difficult to achieve. Also, if the patient works during the night and sleeps during the daytime, he may need to be advised regarding the antihypertensive medications daily schedule.

Determining the patient's *ability to read and understand the literature* that he is given about hypertension, its complications, and treatment is important. Also the ability to communicate and ask questions must be evaluated.

It is not unusual for hypertension to be first detected during *pregnancy.* If hypertension appears during one or more pregnancies and disappears in between, there is less risk than if the hypertension persists between pregnancies. Severe hypertension is a relative contraindication to pregnancy, and if the patient already has children, it may be advisable not to undergo further pregnancies.

The *date of the last menstrual period* helps determine if the patient is pregnant when first seen. Also urinalysis may show blood if the patient is menstruating at the time urine is collected. In that case, no other cause for blood in the urine need be looked for. *Oral contraceptives* can cause hypertension, and it is therefore important to determine if the patient is presently taking oral contraceptives or has received them in the past.

All *medications* being taken by the patient are recorded. A patient may already be taking a diuretic for weight loss and still have hypertension. This would indicate to the physician that a diuretic alone may not be enough for hypertension control. On the other hand, the patient may be taking an anorexic agent for weight loss. Most anorexants are related to amphetamines, which cause vasoconstriction and thus may contribute to hypertension. The patient may be taking nonprescription preparations for a cold or sinus condition, which are sympathetic stimulators and may contribute toward hypertension.

Allergies such as asthma and serious sinus conditions are also recorded, since these are contraindications to propranolol therapy. Also, any allergies to other medications, including antihypertensives, should be indicated.

Any other salient history not already recorded should also be noted.

PHYSICAL EXAMINATION

The patient's *general appearance* is noted, particularly in relation to the patient's gait, coordination, and speech. Hirsutism and truncal obesity are indications of Cushing's syndrome. *Weight, height, and body frame* are recorded and compared with standard charts to see if the patient is overweight or obese. The body frame is judged by having the patient hold his left wrist between the right thumb and the index. If the tips of the fingers touch, the patient has a medium frame; if they do not, he has a large frame; and if they overlap, a small frame. *Pulse rate* and regularity should then be noted. *Peripheral pulses*, that is, the radial, carotid, and femoral pulses, are palpated. A weak pulse or presence of a bruit over it indicates the presence of arteriosclerosis.

At the time of the first visit, the *blood pressure* should be recorded in both arms and a note made as to which side is higher. A discrepancy of up to 5 mm. Hg is not unusual. However, a larger difference may indicate the narrowing of an artery on the side the blood pressure is lower. On follow-up visits the blood pressure is always recorded on the side with the higher blood pressure.

A larger cuff should be used for obese people. The rubber bladder of the blood pressure cuff should have a width equal to one third to one half the length of the upper arm and a length equal to at least two thirds of its circumference. The arm with the cuff wrapped around it is placed at the level of the heart so that hydrostatic pressure does not alter the blood pressure reading. Details of blood pressure measurement are described in Chapter 8. Leg blood pressure is recorded by wrapping a leg cuff around the thigh and auscultating over the popliteal artery, with the patient preferably lying prone. Leg blood pressure should be recorded routinely in children and adolescents with hypertension and in adults who have a delayed or weak femoral pulsation.

The *fundi* are examined in a dark room with the patient looking straight at a distant point. The hypertensive retinopathy is graded from i to iv in increasing severity. Grade i signifies the presence of arterial narrowing or spasm; grade ii, the presence of arteriovenous nicking; grade iii, the presence of hemorrhages and exudates; and grade iv, the presence of papilledema. Grades iii and iv are considered indicative of accelerated and malignant hypertension, respectively.

The *neck* is examined for the presence of goiter or any other swelling. A note is made if the jugular veins are prominent and distended.

The *cardiac examination* consists of palpating the point of maximal impulse (PMI, or apex beat), which is shifted downward and laterally as the heart enlarges. Auscultation is then performed for rhythm, heart sounds, and the presence of murmurs. As indicated in Chapter 1, an S_4 sound indicates a rigid left ventricle due to left ventricular hypertrophy, and an S_3 sound is an early sign of congestive heart failure.

The *lungs* are then auscultated for the presence of rales or wheezing. Basal rales are present in congestive heart failure. Wheezing may indicate heart failure, chronic bronchitis, or asthma.

The *abdomen* is inspected and palpated to determine the presence of enlarged kidneys. Polycystic kidneys and grossly enlarged hydronephrotic kidneys are generally easily palpable. Careful auscultation over the epigastrium will usually reveal a continuous bruit in patients with renal artery stenosis. It is not uncommon to hear a systolic bruit in the epigastrium, particularly in older patients. This is produced by the flow of blood through the celiac artery and is of no significance.

The *legs* are then examined for the presence of edema and signs of peripheral vascular disease such as discoloration of the skin, loss of temperature, or absence of dorsalis pedis pulsations. The skin should be closely inspected for neurofibromatosis and café au lait spots, which are often seen in patients with pheochromocytoma.

A *neurologic examination* for muscle strength and deep tendon reflexes is performed to detect the presence of stroke, of which the patient may or may not be aware.

The *prostate* is examined in older males. Enlarged prostate and urinary retention may cause kidney damage, which can lead to or contribute toward hypertension.

LABORATORY INVESTIGATIONS[1]

Certain laboratory investigations are routinely performed as part of the evaluation of a hypertensive patient.

Urinalysis is necessary, since proteinuria usually indicates renal disease and hypertension may be secondary to the renal parenchymal disease. However, long-standing hypertension can cause nephrosclerosis, ischemic glomerulopathy, and mild to moderate proteinuria.

Glycosuria can be easily diagnosed with dipstick urinalysis. Almost 10% of hypertensives have diabetes. The presence of occult blood may indicate a renal or urinary tract disorder. A microscopic examination of the urine must always be undertaken if the dipstick urinalysis is abnormal (presence of protein or blood). This helps determine the nature of renal disease. The presence of red blood cell casts are pathognomonic of glomerulonephritis. However, granular casts simply indicate the presence of a renal disease.

It is a good practice to routinely record the patient's *hematocrit* before undertaking treatment of hypertension. Many hypertensives tend to have a somewhat higher hematocrit level. It is possible that these patients have high blood viscosity and may be benefited by regular blood donations. If the patient is anemic, he may be dizzy from anemia rather than hypertension.

Fasting blood sugar or a 2-hour postprandial blood sugar measurement should be done for the diagnosis of diabetes. Since blood lipids are drawn in a fasting state, we perform only a fasting blood sugar measurement. As indicated before, the diuretic therapy can cause slight but significant elevations in fasting blood sugar levels and may produce glycosuria in patients who otherwise have only mild elevations in blood sugar.

BUN or *creatinine* elevation indicates renal insufficiency, which may be either the cause or the result of hypertension. A slight rise in BUN can be expected to occur after diuretic therapy. If BUN is normal, it is usually not necessary to measure creatinine. However, if BUN is elevated, serum creatinine should always be measured because it is a more accurate indicator of renal dysfunction.

Serum potassium measurement is an excellent screening measure for primary aldosteronism. A normal serum potassium (3.5 to 5 mEq.) on a normal diet excludes primary aldosteronism for all practical purposes. Serum potassium can be expected to drop by 0.5 to 1.5 mEq. with diuretic therapy. However, in most patients receiving less than 50 mg. hydrochlorothiazide or an equivalent dose of another diuretic, hypokalemia is not a problem.

Serum cholesterol and triglyceride measurements are done to determine the presence of other risk factors such as hypercholesterolemia. After prolonged diuretic therapy, serum lipids may show slight elevation.

Uric acid measurement is not essential for evaluation or to determine the presence of a risk factor; however, the uric acid level does rise with diuretic therapy, and some patients may develop clinical gout. If the uric acid level is more than 10 mg./dl., initiation of prophylactic hypouricemic therapy may be advisable.

Serum calcium measurement is useful in determining the presence of hyperparathyroidism, which can cause hypertension. Also serum calcium level rises with diuretic therapy.

Electrocardiogram (ECG) should be done routinely in patients 40 years of age or older and in younger patients with severe hypertension (diastolic BP $\geq$ 120 mm. Hg), cardiac symptoms, arrhythmias, or a strong family history of heart disease. Evidence of left ventricular hypertrophy or myocardial ischemia are signs of hypertensive cardiovascular disease.

Chest x-ray examination is done primarily to determine the heart size and presence of congestive heart failure. Since clinical symptoms and signs·along with ECG are much better indicators in this regard, we routinely perform a chest x-ray examination only in patients over 60 years of age. If signs of heart failure are present and ECG is abnormal, a chest x-ray examination is a useful way to monitor the patient's condition.

SPECIAL INVESTIGATIONS[2]

After the initial evaluation, if a patient is suspected to have secondary hypertension, appropriate laboratory and radiologic investigations are undertaken to prove or disprove the suspected diagnosis. It is fruitless to investigate a patient for all possible causes of secondary hypertension. Only those investigations need be carried out that would help in the diagnosis of a certain suspected cause of secondary hypertension.

Renal hypertension

Kidney disease is suspected as a cause of hypertension on the basis of history of kidney disease, urinary tract infections, family history of uremia, presence of palpable kidneys, abnormal urinalysis, or elevated serum creatinine.

The diagnosis is supported by intravenous pyelography. If the serum creatinine level is elevated, an infusion urogram better delineates the kidneys and urinary tract. If one kidney is dysplastic or nonfunctioning, split renal vein renin studies and renal angiography are necessary to confirm a diagnosis of renal hypertension. The renal vein renin level on the abnormal side is usually 1.5 to two times the opposite kidney. If the diagnosis is not obvious from blood tests and radiographic studies, renal biopsy may be undertaken to make a specific diagnosis. Renal biopsy should never be taken lightly and should only be done by an experienced nephrologist. The tissues are examined by light, electron, and immunofluorescence microscopy, all three being necessary for an accurate diagnosis.

Renal artery stenosis

Renal artery stenosis occurs most commonly as a result of fibromuscular hyperplasia or atherosclerotic narrowing of one or both renal arteries. The incidence of fibromuscular hyperplasia is greatest in white women under the age of 50 years. Atherosclerotic renovascular hypertension usually occurs after the age of 50 years. The diagnosis should be suspected in patients who have a continuous epigastric bruit, which often radiates to the side of the lesion, or if the patient has severe hypertension that has not responded to treatment.

The diagnosis is confirmed by a rapid-sequence (hypertensive) intravenous pyelography. This is obtained by taking films at 1-minute intervals after the injection of the urographic contrast material. A difference of more than 1.5 cm. in kidney size, delayed appearance of the contrast medium at 1 minute or more on one side, unilateral hyperconcentration of the medium in a 10- to 20-minute film, and ureteral and renal pelvic notching because of collateral circulation are common findings in cases with renal artery stenosis. [131]I Hippuran renogram can further help confirm the diagnosis of renovascular lesion. Renal vein renin measurements and renal angiography are then undertaken for the final confirmation of the diagnosis. The renal vein renin level on the side of the lesion is 1.5 to two times the opposite. Fibromuscular hyperplasia typically has a beaded appearance on angiography. Renal atherosclerotic lesion is typically at the origin of the renal artery.

Primary aldosteronism

Primary aldosteronism is more frequent in young white females. The diagnosis should be suspected if the patient complains of symptoms suggestive of hypokalemia such as muscle weakness, fatigue, polyuria, and nocturia. The serum potassium is usually less than 3.5 mEq./liter in untreated patients or less than 2.5 mEq./liter in those receiving diuretics. Metabolic alkalosis is frequently present, and the urinary potassium excretion even in the presence of hypokalemia generally exceeds 40 mEq./24 hr.

The diagnosis is suspected further by measurement of peripheral plasma renin activity after 2 to 3 days of a low-salt diet (sodium, 10 mEq./24 hr.), furosemide (40 mg. daily for 2 to 3 days) therapy, and 3 to 4 hours of ambulation. The plasma renin activity is either low or undetectable. Increased 24-hour urinary aldosterone (normal range is 4 to 20 μg./24 hr.) is helpful in further confirmation of the diagnosis. This is more reliable than an isolated measurement of plasma aldosterone (normal range is 5 to 12 ng./dl.). For localization of the lesion, adrenal venography and measurement of adrenal venous aldosterone levels are helpful.

Cushing's syndrome

Cushing's syndrome is suspected if the patient has hypertension, truncal obesity, deposition of fat on the nape of the neck, pigmented striae on the abdomen, proximal weakness of muscles, and hyperglycemia. Hirsutism may also be present. The diagnosis is confirmed by measurement of plasma cortisol at 8 A.M. and 4 P.M. Patients with Cushing's syndrome almost always have plasma cortisol in excess of 15 μg./ml. In normal subjects, in response to 1 mg. dexamethasone given at 11 P.M. the previous night, the plasma cortisol secretion is suppressed. Patients with Cushing's syndrome always maintain increased secretion of cortisol. ACTH level determination will help decide whether the hypercorticism is primary or secondary to ACTH stimulation.

Pheochromocytoma

Pheochromocytoma is suspected if the patient complains of paroxysmal episodes of headache, flushing (or pallor), sweating, and/or palpitations. Between episodes the hypertension may be mild or absent, but during an episode the blood pressure is usually severely elevated. The patient may have experienced symptoms of orthostatic hypotension, and diastolic blood pressure may fall when the patient stands up. Multiple neurofibromas, café au lait spots, or a palpable thyroid mass may be present.

The diagnosis is confirmed by a 24-hour urinary assay for total catecholamines, metanephrines, and vanillylmandelic acid (VMA). Pharmacologic tests using phentolamine and glucagon were used in the past but are less reliable and somewhat dangerous. Selective adrenal artery angiograms are helpful in localizing the tumor but should be done only by an experienced radiologist, since the test can bring about release of adrenalin and precipitate severe hypertensive crisis.

Coarctation of aorta

Coarctation of the aorta is suspected if the patient complains of cold feet, claudication, or both; femoral pulses are weak or absent, and blood pressures recorded over the popliteal artery is lower than in the brachial artery. An extra cardiac murmur is often present in the precordial area. Although the chest x-ray film may show rib notching due to collateral arteries and a poststenotic dilation of the aorta, aortogram is necessary for confirmation and exact localization of the coarctation.

Miscellaneous causes of secondary hypertension

Causes of secondary hypertension include 17-hydroxylase deficiency in which cortisol secretion is low and aldosterone secretion is high, acute porphyria, acute lead intoxication, and raised intracranial tension. Appropriate tests can be undertaken to confirm these diagnoses.

SUMMARY

The purpose of evaluation of hypertensive patients is not only to diagnose secondary hypertension when present but also to detect the presence of other risk factors and evidence of damage to the blood vessels, heart, brain, and kidneys. Also evaluated are patients' personal habits and attitudes toward their health.

The history is the most important and time-consuming part of the evaluation. The physical examination is tailored to detect signs of secondary hypertension and the extent of target organ damage. Laboratory investigations consist of urinalysis and other tests that help in detection of certain causes of secondary hypertension and provide information on patient's general health. ECG is useful in detecting left ventricular hypertrophy, which develops earlier than cardiac dilation. Cardiac dilation is best seen on the chest x-ray film. Not every hypertensive needs these investigations.

Further investigations, which include x-ray examination and biochemical tests, are undertaken when a particular cause of secondary hypertension is suspected. Only those investigations are necessary that would help in the diagnosis of the suspected condition.

SUGGESTED READINGS

1. Beeson, P. B., and McDermott, W.: Textbook of medicine, ed. 14, Philadelphia, 1975, W. B. Saunders Co.
2. Kaplan, N. M.: Clinical hypertension, New York, 1973, Medcom Press.

CHAPTER **5**

Treatment of hypertension

Nurses are beginning to address the problem of hypertension more aggresive-ly by expanding their role in community and patient education and by focusing on the detection and monitoring of hypertensive individuals. Nurse-managed hypertension clinics that operate within the framework of standardized protocols have been developed and are proving successful. This approach provides more comprehensive and beneficial services to the patient and family such as relating to one professional team, individualized educational services, and continuous motivation and support. This allows the physician more time to care for the acutely and critically ill patients. Without the help of nurses and other allied health professionals, it would be impossible for the limited number of physicians to provide care for the estimated 35 to 50 million hypertensives in the United States. The nurse benefits from the satisfaction and enjoyment of providing qual-ity ambulatory nursing care through an expanded role. In addition, it gives her the stimulating independence necessary for further development and research in patient care services.

TREATMENT OF ESSENTIAL HYPERTENSION

Our operational philosophy is to control hypertension and prevent compli-cations in the simplest, safest, most effective, and most individualized manner possible. Consistent with this philosophy and recently employed as therapy for hypertension is the use of *behavioral methods.* These include biofeedback,[2] relaxation, psychotherapy, suggestion, and environmental modification. The reasoning behind the use of these methods is that emotional events in the life of an individual influence one's blood pressure and affect the course of hypertension.

Biofeedback employs modern instrumentation which gives an individual moment-to-moment feedback about a specific physiologic process that is regulated by the autonomic nervous system but that is not consciously perceived and controlled. One can be trained to develop control over the physiologic process. Use of biofeedback in control of hypertension is still in early experimental stages. Blood pressure falls ranging up to 20/10 mm. Hg have been reported.

Relaxation methods such as *yoga, transcendental meditation,* and the *relaxation response* have been proposed for the treatment of hypertension. They seek to elicit calmness and a hypometabolic state associated with decreased sympathetic activity and lowering of blood pressure. They have been practiced for hundreds of years in India and other eastern countries and were not specifically devised for the treatment of hypertension. Reported reductions in blood pressure have a wide range, from 7/4 mm. Hg to 37/22 mm. Hg. Transcendental meditation and the relaxation response are relatively easy to learn, and their use should be encouraged if the patient is so inclined.

Traditional *verbal psychotherapy* as a method of lowering blood pressure has been proposed because of the relief that it can provide to anxious individuals and as an aid to hypertensive patients in dealing with aggressive and hostile impulses. Declines in blood pressure up to 20 to 40 mm. Hg systolic and 10 to 30 mm. Hg diastolic may be achieved with continued therapy. Supportive therapy in the form of patient counseling is always recommended because it augments compliance. Analytic psychotherapy is expensive and time-consuming and should be used only when indicated on the basis of a patient's psychiatric need independent of hypertension.

Suggestion as a therapeutic measure has been moderately successful, with blood pressure reductions of 15/10 mm. Hg. Based on this success, before recording blood pressure, the patient should always be asked to relax and be comfortable.

Environmental modification to lower blood pressure is based on the hypothesis that stressful stimuli arising in an individual's environment adversely affect one's blood pressure. However, with the exception of hospitalization, environmental manipulation as therapy for hypertension has not been shown to have salutary effect on hypertension.

Control of obesity, smoking, and salt intake are appropriate adjunct modes helpful in management of hypertension and are discussed in detail in Chapter 6.

The behavioral methods just discussed are not yet in widespread use. They seem to be useful adjuncts and not alternative methods to the drug treatment of essential hypertension.

DRUG THERAPY

Antihypertensive medications are the mainstay of treatment of hypertension. The results of the Veterans Administration Cooperative Study previously referred to in Chapter 1 indicate that drug treatment of hypertension reduces morbidity and mortality in patients with diastolic pressures of 105 mm. Hg or higher. The first goal of antihypertensive therapy is to achieve and maintain diastolic pressure levels at less than 90 mm. Hg. This can be accomplished in more than 85% of hypertensive patients with minimal adverse effects regardless of the initial severity of the disease.

Stepped-care approach

Antihypertensive therapy is initiated with a small dose of an antihypertensive drug. The dose is increased and other drugs are added to achieve the predetermined level of blood pressure. Monitoring and evaluation at regular intervals are necessary, with alterations either up or down the steps as warranted. Moving down the steps if possible while maintaining adequate blood pressure control is of course desirable.

Our stepped-care approach based on the recommendations of the Joint National Committee on Detection, Evaluation, and Treatment of High Blood Pressure[1] is as follows:

Step I   Diuretics
Step II Add reserpine, methyldopa, propranolol, prazosin, or clonidine
Step III Add prazosin or hydralazine
Step IV Add or substitute guanethidine

The first step should ordinarily be a thiazide-type diuretic. There is no demonstrable advantage of a long-acting diuretic such as chlorthalidone or a short-acting loop diuretic such as furosemide over hydrochlorothiazide in terms of antihypertensive effect. Dietary supplements are usually sufficient to prevent hypokalemia.

If the therapeutic goal is not achieved with the diuretic alone, consideration is given to adding a step II drug. Any one of the five drugs mentioned can be used. Diuretic therapy must always be continued. Whichever drug is chosen, it is first administered in small dosages and increased gradually until the therapeutic effect is achieved, side effects develop, or maximum recommended dose is reached. Reversal of antihypertensive effect after initial response may indicate fluid retention, requiring an increase in the dose of the diuretic. In most instances, there is little advantage in substituting one step II drug for another. Substitution is indicated if the patient is unable to tolerate a certain step II drug.

When a third drug is needed, prazosin or hydralazine may be added to the regimen. Both are effective peripheral vasodilators. The reflex tachycardia with prazosin is less than with hydralazine.

Addition or substitution of guanethidine may be necessary if the first three steps of the regimen are ineffective and the causes for unresponsiveness have been investigated. These patients require more careful follow-up.

Antihypertensive drug protocol

The present protocol for stepped-care treatment of hypertension in our clinic is as follows:

1. Start the antihypertensive therapy with 25 mg./24 hr. hydrochlorothiazide. Increase the dose to 50 mg./24 hr.
2. Switch to Aldoril-25 (methyldopa, 250 mg. and hydrochlorothiazide, 25 mg.), one tablet daily. Increase to twice daily.
3. Substitute Aldoril-15 (methyldopa, 250 mg., and hydrochlorothiazide, 15 mg.), two tablets in the morning and one tablet in the evening. Increase to two tablets twice daily.
4. Add prazosin, 1 mg., twice daily. Increase at weekly intervals to 2, 4, 5, and 10 mg. twice daily as necessary.
5. Switch to Ser-Ap-Es (reserpine, 0.1 mg.; hydralazine, 25 mg.; and hydrochlorothiazide, 15 mg.), one tablet twice daily. Increase the dose to six tablets daily.
6. Administer hydrochlorothiazide, 50 mg./24 hr., and increasing doses of guanethidine, starting at 10 mg./24 hr. Add hydralazine, 25 mg., twice daily and increase the dose until the patient is receiving a maximum of 100 mg./24 hr. hydrochlorothiazide, 100 mg./24 hr. guanethidine, and 200 mg./24 hr. hydralazine.
7. Try other antihypertensives including phenoxybenzamine in rational combinations.

Utilizing combination tablets for antihypertensive therapy has positive as well as negative factors. One advantage of combination tablets is that patients' adherence to drug therapy is improved because most patients find multiple pills in multiple doses confusing. Frequently, combination tablets are less expensive than the same regimen administered in separate tablets. The problems arise with the clinician's inability to adjust the dosage of each ingredient separately. Occasionally this individualization of dosage is necessary for successful blood pressure control. Additionally, the trade names can be confusing to both patient and clinician, and the possibility exists that the patient may receive inappropriate dosages or combinations of drugs. If the hypertension is refractory and presents considerable problems with control requiring frequent dose adjustment, combination tablets are not recommended. Once control is achieved, combination tablets, if found in the right dose proportion, are then employed.

Although there are many possible effective therapeutic regimens, we follow the previous protocol because it has proved effective in lowering blood pressure and is well tolerated by patients. We use combination pills and administer antihypertensives on a twice daily regimen to promote compliance.

Pretreatment considerations

Attention needs to be paid to drug sensitivities. Patients allergic to sulfa drugs may also be allergic to thiazide diuretics because of chemical similarity. The patient may have been previously treated with certain antihypertensives and found to be allergic to one or more of them. These agents should not be administered again. Contraindications to the use of certain antihypertensives may be present. For example, methyldopa is contraindicated in patients with liver dysfunction and propranolol in asthmatics.

Drug interaction is another factor that can significantly affect the patient. Tricyclic antidepressants such as amitriptyline (Elavil) and others displace guanethidine from the adrenergic nerve endings, thus reversing its effect. The decongestants contain ephedrine-like compounds that produce vasoconstriction and can interfere with antihypertensive therapy.

Classification of hypertensive patients and treatment schemes

Although all patients must receive individualized therapy programs, it is helpful to classify the patient according to the severity of hypertension as it helps in selecting appropriate initial antihypertensive therapy. We classify them as follows:

Age	Mild	Moderate	Severe
18-49 years	140/90-154/104 mm. Hg	155/105-169/119 mm. Hg	≥170/120 mm. Hg
50-59 years	150/95-164/104 mm. Hg	165/105-179/119 mm. Hg	≥180/120 mm. Hg
≥60 years	160/95-174/104 mm. Hg	175/105-189/119 mm. Hg	≥190/120 mm. Hg

At the initial evaluation, 10% of our untreated hypertensive patients have labile hypertension; 42%, mild; 24%, moderate; and 24%, severe. We use the following treatment schemes, depending on the initial blood pressure.

Labile hypertension. Drug therapy for individuals with labile hypertension is highly individualized. The patient needs to be thoroughly evaluated with careful consideration of cardiovascular risk factors. If a decision is made to delay the drug therapy, the patient is monitored on a 3- to 6-month basis with a risk factor modification program. There is no clear data at this time to validate zealous drug therapy in these patients. Certainly the chances of developing essential hypertension later are increased, and continued observation is indicated. Salt restriction, behavioral methods of blood pressure reduction, exercise, and weight control are helpful in maintaining blood pressure at a reasonable level. Drug therapy is initiated if the patient continues to have periods of severe hypertension, although the hypertension remains labile. Other indications for drug therapy are strong family history of hypertension or the presence of hypertensive complications or the presence of other cardiovascular risk factors.

Mild hypertension. Treatment of patients with diastolic pressure from 90 to 104 mm. Hg is again individualized. Weight control and reduced salt intake may lower blood pressure in some individuals. The presence of the following factors in a patient with mild diastolic hypertension influences the decision to begin drug treatment:

- Elevated systolic blood pressure
- Hypertensive retinopathy or other evidence of arteriosclerosis
- Left ventricular hypertrophy
- Strong family history of hypertension
- Other cardiovascular risk factors such as heavy smoking, high serum cholesterol, diabetes, heavy drinking, or obesity
- Black race and male sex

Certain patients with mild hypertension request that drug therapy be postponed. These patients are encouraged to pursue a low-salt diet, lose weight as necessary, and perhaps practice relaxation techniques, attempting to lower blood pressure. After a 3-month monitoring period, the patient is again evaluated, and if still hypertensive, drug therapy is initiated. If the blood pressure is normal, nonpharmacologic therapy is continued, but the patient is still monitored at 3-month intervals, similar to those treated with medications.

Moderate hypertension. Patients with diastolic levels of 105 to 119 mm. Hg, which is within the moderate range of hypertension, definitely require treatment. In these patients with uncomplicated hypertension, risk factor modifications and diuretic agents are the first step. If after a month the blood pressure is not controlled, the patient is advanced progressively through steps of the protocol on a monthly basis until the blood pressure is controlled.

Patients with moderate elevations and complications such as angina, symptoms of congestive heart failure, cardiomegaly, previous myocardial infarction, peripheral vascular or retinal changes, proteinuria, or slightly elevated serum creatinine ($\geq$2 mg./dl.) are initiated on treatment with a full diuretic dosage in combination with methyldopa. The physician monitors these patients on a weekly to biweekly basis until blood pressure control is achieved and complications improve. Additional investigations, evaluation, and treatment of complications are performed as indicated.

Severe hypertension. Hypertensive patients with diastolic blood pressure $\geq$120 mm. Hg require prompt antihypertensive therapy. Treatment is usually started at step II and the patient followed weekly until hypertension control is achieved and complications are improved.

Management of hypertensive patients with diastolic blood pressure of 130 mm. Hg or higher is discussed in the section on hypertensive emergencies.

Monitoring therapy

The following parameters are utilized in monitoring patients during follow-up visits:

1. Blood pressure level
2. Drug therapy compliance
3. Symptoms, adverse side effects, complications, and laboratory data

If the blood pressure is controlled and the patient feels well, the medication is continued as previously prescribed. If the blood pressure is below 120/80 mm. Hg, the medication is decreased one step on the protocol. For example, if a 25-year-old patient has a blood pressure of 110/70 mm. Hg, is asymptomatic, and is taking 50 mg. hydrochlorothiazide once daily, the dosage can be decreased to 25 mg. once daily. If the patient is taking 25 mg. hydrochlorothiazide once a day, is asymptomatic, and has a blood pressure of 110/70 mm. Hg, the medication can be decreased to every other day. Finally, if the patient is taking hydrochlorothiazide every other day with a blood pressure of 110/70 mm. Hg, the medication can be discontinued; however, the patient should be monitored on a 3- to 6-month basis for the duration of his life.

If the blood pressure is elevated, the medication can be advanced one step on the protocol. This action requires a more comprehensive evaluation of current patient status. Consideration must be given to the anxiety level of the patient. The blood pressure is always measured on the same arm that originally gave the highest reading and is repeated after the patient has rested a short time. Other factors such as smoking, cold, and stress are considered for possible blood pressure elevating effects.

An accurate assessment of drug compliance is essential. We request patients to bring all current medications in their containers. A rough estimate of adherence to the drug regimen by comparing pills prescribed with pills remaining can be easily done. In addition, thorough questioning regarding drug compliance as presented in Chapter 7 is attempted. If noncompliance is suspected, the medication may be continued as previously prescribed, with an assessment to determine the cause of noncompliance and strategies to motivate compliance initiated. Strong advice emphasizing the need and rationale for drug therapy, and reinforcement with clarification of the problem of hypertension and its complications should be provided. An individualized, personalized, and caring approach does work. The patient is shown his record of blood pressure, weight, pulse, smoking and diet habits, and laboratory data to demonstrate his personal progress, with the emphasis placed on increasing his responsibility for his body and his life (i.e., the health care professonals are sending the message, "We care and we want you to care and take care"). Appealing to personal and rational patient aspects further cements the therapeutic contract.

If the patient does take the medications as prescribed and the blood pressure is still elevated, an increase in salt content of the diet is suspected. This can raise the blood pressure by 10/5 mm. Hg. If indicated after questioning, further counseling to promote compliance with salt intake modification is provided.

Drug antagonism by the patient's use of competing drugs such as over-the-counter cold remedies should be evaluated. With regard to female patients, the clinician must ask whether they have started taking birth control pills or, if meno-pausal, whether estrogen replacement was started by the patient's gynecologist.

Another consideration the clinician should evaluate in drug therapy failure is insufficient control of plasma volume through inadequate diuretic therapy. If dietary modification of salt intake and medication compliance is assured, higher dosages of diuretics would then be warranted. Finally, the presence of secondary hypertension must be considered. This is discussed later in the chapter.

The suggested time schedule for return visits is presented in the box on p. 69.

Home monitoring of blood pressure is a useful way to determine hypertension control. This can be an important tool for patient participation in the therapeutic plan to control hypertension and to characterize the blood pressure readings on a daily basis under more normal circumstances. If the patient is willing, we en-courage use of this method and provide training. We suggest a weekly recording of blood pressure. If possible, it should be recorded in the same arm and at the same time of day in a comfortable sitting posture. This is undertaken when the patient's blood pressure has stabilized and he has had the benefit of an extensive hypertension counseling program. The patient is taught the theory and tech-nique of blood pressure measurement similar to the volunteer training program described in Chapter 8. Repeated practice sessions are conducted. A daily graph can be devised. With this basis, the patient is instructed not to alter medication dose or frequency. If any questions or problems arise, the patient is requested to call the clinic. His blood pressure instrument is returned to the clinic periodi-cally for accuracy and a maintenance check. A "track record" of blood pressure is generally more valuable than a single office blood pressure level measurement in determining whether the blood pressure is controlled. If a patient is too appre-hensive about his elevated blood pressure, we discourage home blood pressure measurement.

Dealing with common side effects

Side effects need to be anticipated with drug therapy. More often than not, they are mild to moderate in degree and diminish with time, which can be a few days to a few months. Certain side effects are relatively common and are sec-ondary results of the drugs preferred action. A discussion of side effects common to many antihypertensives follows.

Dry mouth and frequent voiding. These side effects occur with diuretic therapy. As diuretics increase the urine output, the plasma volume is reduced, resulting in a state of mild dehydration and causing dryness of the mouth. Most patients tolerate this well. For others, simple measures such as chewing a sugar-less candy or gum is recommended. Some patients find it too inconvenient to void frequently during working hours. Furosemide can be prescribed to be taken on returning home from work. The diuretic action of this drug lasts less than 4 hours. Despite continued diuretic therapy, eventually plasma volume returns to near normal in most patients and they cease to experience dryness of mouth

FREQUENCY OF CLINIC VISITS

Patient diagnosis and protocol status	Suggested intervals between clinic visits
Labile or mild hypertension	
Risk factor modification and blood pressure monitoring	3 months
Diuretic therapy initiated	1 month
Controlled on diuretic therapy	3 months
Moderate hypertension	
Diuretic therapy initiated (no complications)	1 month
Controlled on diuretic therapy (no complications)	3 months
Not controlled on step II antihypertensives (no complications)	1 month
Controlled on step II antihypertensives (no complications)	3 months
Not controlled on step II antihypertensives and/or complications present	Individualized: weekly, biweekly, or monthly
Severe hypertension	
Not controlled—step II antihypertensives initiated (no complications)	1 month
Controlled on step II antihypertensives (no complications)	3 months
Not controlled on step II; step III antihypertensives initiated (no complications)	Individualized: weekly, biweekly, or monthly
Controlled on step III antihypertensives (no complications)	3 months
Controlled on step III antihypertensives (hypertensive or drug therapy complications present)	Individualized: weekly, biweekly, or monthly
Not controlled on step III antihypertensive or hypertensive or drug therapy complications present	Individualized: weekly, biweekly, or monthly. Hospitalization may be necessary

and urinary frequency. An important consideration is that diuretics can induce diabetes. Therefore the urine should be screened for sugar and acetone if the symptoms persist.

Fatigue, lethargy, and drowsiness. As their blood pressure falls, many patients develop one or more of these symptoms, with the usual expression being, "I don't have as much pep." Almost all antihypertensive drugs can cause fatigue, lethargy, and drowsiness, methyldopa and clonidine probably more than others. Serum potassium can be measured to rule out diuretic-induced hypokalemia and liver enzymes assessed to exclude methyldopa-induced liver damage. If no cause for the symptoms is determined, the patient may be reassured that the symptoms will be temporary and will disappear as the body adapts to the lower blood pressure and the effects of drugs. If the symptoms are intolerable and/or persist beyond 3 months, alternate antihypertensives may be prescribed. The patient also must be advised to employ caution during driving or operating machinery.

Dizziness and lightheadedness. These symptoms are indicative of orthostatic hypotension. They are not uncommon when the patient first receives sympathetic inhibitors, methyldopa, or guanethidine. The patient can be warned to avoid hot weather, strenuous exercise, and alcohol consumption within 3 hours of taking medications. To prevent the postural dizziness and faintness, the patient is given the following advice:

1. Slow down body movements; for example, when arising from bed in the morning, first sit up at the side of the bed for a few moments. When comfortable, begin to stand slowly. Generally, the body will signal if it is moving too fast by beginning to feel weak or faint. With movement the dizziness usually disappears.
2. Wear support stockings, which can be put on before getting up from bed in the morning. This keeps the blood from collecting in the legs.
3. Sleep with the head of the bed raised about 6 inches with pillows or blocks so that the posture change is minimized after awakening.
4. Lie down and rest awhile until the faintness passes and then slowly begin moving again.
5. Avoid operating heavy machinery or driving.
6. Be patient with oneself.

The blood pressure needs to be measured in the supine and standing positions to evaluate the presence and degree of hypotensive changes. If this continues to be a significant problem, consideration may be given to altering medication schedules, such as taking the drug in the evening or before sleep. In addition, the strength of the dose may be divided differently. If methyldopa (Aldomet), 500 mg. once a day, is prescribed, consider 250 mg. twice a day.

If the aforementioned nursing suggestions are to no avail and postural hypotension still persists, the dose of the drug most likely responsible for the symptoms should be reduced. If symptoms still persist, consideration should be given to switching to another drug.

Thus the nurse's role is to obtain an accurate history, to provide detailed anticipatory guidance for the prevention and management of orthostatic hypotension, and specifically to assess this problem at each encounter.

Sexual dysfunction. Loss of libido and impotence are side effects of sympathetic inhibitor and vasodilator therapy. These problems may be more prevalent than generally voiced by the patients. This may be an unstated reason for drug noncompliance. Normal autonomic function is essential for erection and ejaculation. Erection is more dependent on the parasympathetic nervous system, whereas orgasm and ejaculation are more dependent on the sympathetic nervous system. Hence the sympathetic inhibitors primarily affect the orgasm and ejaculation. The ejaculation may be either delayed or the orgasm less intense. Sometimes with high doses of guanethidine, the ejaculation may occur retrograde or into the bladder, since the sphincter muscle at the bladder neck does not fully close. This can be worrisome for some patients, but if explained properly, many patients tolerate this dysfunction well.

It is our impression that sexual dysfunction may be related to the lowering of blood pressure regardless of the medications used. Elevated blood pressure may increase potency by a greater pressure head causing a greater and stronger erection. When blood pressure is lowered and sexual function returns to "normal," the patient may perceive this as impotence. In our opinion this is the mechanism of impotence in some patients; certain individuals have complained of impotence after their blood pressure was lowered with nonpharmacologic means, such as weight reduction, low-salt diet, or diuretic therapy alone. Once again, if the patient is provided with the explanation that it is normal to experience some "slowing down" as the blood pressure is controlled, this problem is well tolerated.

The anticipatory guidance may include the following patient explanations:

> At first, some men may feel changes when having sex. This may be in different ways, like the penis not getting as hard as usual, or not being able to keep the hardness as long as before, or the semen coming out differently. None of these changes are harmful and usually are lessened in time if you relax. You may want to talk this problem over with your partner. This can be very helpful. Being patient with yourself, taking the medicines as ordered, and telling the doctor or nurse about this problem, is what to do.

An open, trusting, and accepting therapeutic relationship will encourage the patient's verbalization of this problem. Phrases often heard that allude to sexual dysfunction include "I'm having trouble with my wife," "My nature is not right," "I can't have sex," and "Can I talk to the doctor about a personal problem, man-to-man?"

The key to management is the patient's perception and tolerance of the problem. Nursing advice involves reassuring and supporting the anxious patient. The nurse can emphasize that this is a temporary effect, possibly due to the lowering of blood pressure and the medication. Stress and nervousness may also contribute. The patient may be reassured by discussing this with the sex partner and by being helped to accept, relax, and be tolerant about this problem.

If these undesirable effects continue and are still perceived as undesirable and threatening, the dosage can be decreased or the drug discontinued. Alternate drugs such as reserpine or hydralazine can be used, but these drugs can also cause impotence. Of hypertensive men maintained on guanethidine, 70% occasionally experience failure of ejaculation, although erection and orgasm are not prevented. Sexual dysfunction in women is less obvious and rarely is a problem.

Weight gain. The physical finding of weight gain by a patient who is on diuretic therapy merits special attention. The nurse must assess the patient's dietary habits to determine whether the weight gain is due to overeating or an increase in salt intake. If it is not, congestive heart failure must be ruled out. A thorough cardiovascular and respiratory physical assessment should be performed. Weight gain associated with lung rales, pedal edema, and/or other symptoms of congestive heart failure warrant immediate physician consultation and management. In addition, the nurse may consider fluid retention as an adverse effect of propranolol, guanethidine, and other sympathetic inhibitors and vasodilator therapy.

Complications of antihypertensive therapy

Complications are adverse effects of antihypertensive drugs distinctly different from the pharmacologic purpose. Although the incidence of side effects is relatively high, severe complications are rare. By means of a thorough history and evaluation, some complications can be anticipated. The patient needs to be appropriately monitored for the onset of complications so that they can be identified and treated immediately. Adverse effects of various antihypertensives are mentioned in Chapter 3. Ways to minimize and reverse them are discussed here.

Diuretics. Hypokalemia (serum potassium < 3.5 mEq./liter) is a well-known complication of diuretic therapy. Many physicians prescribe potassium supplements or potassium-sparing diuretics at the outset to prevent hypokalemia. With a 100 mg./24 hr. dose of hydrochlorothiazide, more than 60% of patients develop serum potassium levels between 3 and 3.5 mEq./liter, but in few cases does the serum potassium level fall below 3 mEq./liter. Since hypokalemic symptoms are unusual unless the serum potassium level falls below 3 mEq./liter, we do not routinely prescribe potassium supplements or potassium-sparing diuretics. The antihypertensive effect of diuretics peaks at a dose equivalent to 50 mg. hydrochlorothiazide. However, the incidence of hypokalemia rises rapidly above that dose. Therefore, we add a step II drug to the diuretic at that point rather than increase the dose of the diuretic.

We routinely encourage our patients to restrict salt, use salt-substitute, and increase the intake of potassium-rich foods, which further reduce the severity and incidence of hypokalemia. Annually and whenever a patient complains of neuromuscular disturbance such as weakness, leg cramps, muscle fatigue, paresthesias, or others or demonstrates hyporeflexia or pulse irregularity, serum potassium is measured. In a symptomatic patient with no other cause for the previous symptoms, a potassium-sparing diuretic is added to the therapeutic regimen even if serum potassium is not low. A combination product such as Aldactazide or Dyazide is preferred to simplify the therapeutic regimen. Our first choice is not potassium supplements, since most taste badly, produce gastrointestinal discomfort, and are generally expensive.

Patients receiving digitalis are routinely prescribed a potassium-sparing diuretic to prevent hypokalemia because digitalis can cause serious arrhythmias in the presence of hypokalemia.

Hyperglycemia is a less commonly encountered complication of diuretics.

Almost all diuretics can cause this complication. The manufacturer of metolazone (Zaroxolyn) suggests a lesser incidence of this complication with their product. The probable mechanisms of diuretic-induced hyperglycemia are inhibition of insulin release from the pancreas and peripheral insulin antagonism. A fasting blood glucose test before initiation of therapy and annually thereafter is recommended. Whenever symptoms suggestive of diabetes develop (polyuria, polyphagia, and polydipsia), the urine and blood must be examined immediately for sugar. If hyperglycemia develops, the patient is advised to restrict carbohydrates and the diabetes appropriately managed. Diuretic therapy is not withdrawn.

Hyperuricemia is a not uncommon complication of diuretic therapy. Serum uric acid measurement is recommended prior to therapy. Hyperuricemia is associated with an increased incidence of gout and urinary tract stones. We routinely prescribe allopurinol (Zyloprim) in patients with pretreatment serum uric acid levels of 10 mg./dl. or more to prevent these complications. Allopurinol is a xanthine oxidase inhibitor and interferes with uric acid synthesis. Generally, 100 mg./24 hr. is sufficient to prevent hyperuricemia. If gout or uric acid stones develop, it is necessary to prescribe 300 mg./24 hr. to prevent their recurrence. Acute gout is treated with indomethacin (Indocin), 25 to 50 mg. three times daily for 4 to 7 days. The serum uric acid level is monitored at least once a year, and allopurinol is prescribed if it rises above 12 mg./dl. on diuretic therapy.

Hypercalcemia is a less commonly encountered complication of thiazide therapy. It does not occur with the use of loop diuretics. Thiazides increase tubular calcium absorption, thus causing serum calcium levels to rise. If persistent hypercalcemia develops ($Ca^{++} \geq 11$ mg./dl.), appropriate investigations need to be undertaken to rule out hyperparathyroidism. If hyperparathyroidism is excluded, the diuretic may be changed to furosemide.

Methyldopa. A number of cases of hemolytic anemia secondary to methyldopa therapy have been reported. It is, however, an uncommon occurrence and in most instances regresses when the drug is discontinued. However, methyldopa is to be avoided in patients with hemolytic anemia due to any cause.

Laboratory evidence of reversible liver damage is not uncommon, and several cases of active chronic hepatitis have been identified. Methyldopa should not be administered to patients with liver dysfunction.

Drug fever, granulocytopenia, and thrombocytopenia are some uncommon allergic complications of methyldopa.

Prazosin. Approximately 1% of patients given 2 mg. or more of prazosin develop syncope within 30 to 90 minutes after the first dose. This adverse effect can be minimized by limiting the initial dose to 1 mg. before sleep and by subsequently increasing the dose slowly. Anticipatory guidance regarding this potential problem is necessary.

Reserpine. Psychic depression is a well-known complication of reserpine. It is therefore contraindicated in patients with a history of depression episodes. If symptoms of depression are manifested, the drug should be discontinued. Since the drug's effects may last 2 weeks or longer, the patient is closely observed.

Reserpine increases gastric acid secretion. It is avoided in patients with peptic ulcer and discontinued if symptoms of peptic ulceration appear. Since reserpine increases appetite and commonly causes weight gain, it is avoided in overweight individuals. Furthermore, if the patient is made aware of this possible effect and provided diet counseling, a weight gain may be avoided.

Increased incidence of carcinoma of the breast in women has been reported with long-term use of reserpine. The drug is avoided in patients with a previous history or family history of malignancy.

Propranolol. Heart failure may develop in patients with inadequate myocardial function.

An increase in airway resistance can be life-threatening in asthmatics. Chronic obstructive pulmonary disease (COPD) is therefore a contraindication to the use of propranolol.

Propranolol augments the hypoglycemic action of insulin by reducing the compensatory effect of adrenalin and is employed cautiously, if at all, in diabetics.

Clonidine. Hyperirritability and a marked rebound in blood pressure due to reversal of the sympathetic blockade can occur in some patients on abrupt withdrawal of clonidine. This results from an increase in catecholamine secretion and can be controlled by adrenergic blockers.

Hydralazine. Long-term hydralazine therapy with 400 mg. or more per day can produce an acute rheumatoid state and a syndrome indistinguishable from disseminated lupus erythematosus. Therefore the dose is limited to 200 mg./24 hr. The symptoms regress after discontinuation of hydralazine. In some patients, long-term steroid therapy may be required.

Guanethidine. Decreased myocardial competence due to decreased adrenergic nerve effects accompanied by fluid accumulation can lead to frank heart failure in patients with compromised cardiac reserve. Such patients are closely monitored for signs of congestive heart failure and treated with digitalis, an increased dose of diuretic, and if necessary withdrawal of guanethidine.

Dealing with ancillary complaints

Many patients with hypertension occasionally have certain nonspecific symptoms that are not directly related to their elevated blood pressure but that must be dealt with. Some common complaints and strategies to deal with them follow.

Headache. Although headache due to hypertension is typically occipital, many hypertensives have frontal or global headache. Normalization of blood pressure only partially relieves it. It is usually a "tension" headache and may be helped by practicing relaxation. It generally responds to either a simple analgesic like acetaminophen (Tylenol, Datril) or aspirin. If these are not sufficient, a combination of acetaminophen and a muscle relaxant such as chlorzoxazone (Parafon Forte) is helpful in relieving headaches in many instances. We avoid the use of potentially habit-forming substances such as propoxyphene (Darvon) and related compounds. If the headache is severe and persistent, further appropriate evaluation and management is undertaken.

Cold. Most OTC cold remedies, because of their decongestant content, carry a label warning that hypertensive patients should avoid taking them. Many hypertensive patients interpret the warning to say that decongestants interact with antihypertensives and that the two should not be taken simultaneously. After catching a cold, they stop the antihypertensive drugs and instead take the cold remedies. We advise our patients to definitely continue taking the antihypertensives and, if necessary, to take the cold remedies in addition. In our experience, pseudoephedrine (Sudafed) causes minimal elevation in blood pressure.

Nervousness and anxiety. Some people are nervous and anxious in dealing with everyday situations. They believe their hypertension is caused by stress. Although the antihypertensive therapy normalizes their blood pressure, they continue to feel anxious. These patients are counseled as described in Chapter 6. If counseling is not sufficient, a benzodiazepine tranquilizer (Librium, Serax, Tranxene, Valium, etc.) is prescribed as necessary. The patient is warned that the drug may be habit-forming and that he needs to use appropriate restraint. Although these minor tranquilizers do not normalize blood pressure, they are useful therapeutic adjuncts in certain patients.

Insomnia. The blood pressure falls during sleep. Although there is no evidence that insomnia leads to hypertension, many patients do have associated insomnia. Appropriate counseling can be provided to determine the cause of insomnia and allay patient's anxieties. In some instances to enhance patient compliance and for total management of a patient's problems, it is necessary to prescribe a sedative. Chloral hydrate (Noctec) and flurazepam (Dalmane) are the drugs most commonly used in our clinic for this purpose because of their relative safety and low potential for addiction.

Chest pain. It is not unusual for a patient to complain of midsternal or precordial discomfort with severe hypertension. The pain is constant, not related to exertion, and generally described as a feeling of "heaviness." The resting ECG is either normal or shows left ventricular hypertrophy without evidence of ischemia. Normalization of blood pressure relieves the symptoms in most instances.

A few patients complain of chest pain that is nonspecific and is not associated with any objective cardiac, esophageal, or pulmonary findings even when appropriately investigated. This pain is usually musculoskeletal in origin. Reassurance helps a great deal, since many patients perceive every chest pain to be of cardiac origin. Use of chlorozoxazone or a similar compound is helpful in relieving the pain.

TREATMENT OF SECONDARY HYPERTENSION

Treatment of secondary hypertension depends on the cause. In some instances, surgical treatment can cure the hypertension. However, in many cases even after the specific cause for hypertension is corrected surgically, blood pressure may remain elevated and require medical therapy.

Renal hypertension

Hypertension in a patient with bilateral renal disease such as glomerulonephritis, polycystic disease, diabetic kidney disease, polyarteritis nodosa, and chronic pyelonephritis requires medical therapy for control of hypertension.

Hypertensive patients with unilateral kidney disease such as dysplastic or a severely traumatized kidney demonstrating minimal or absent renal function in the absence of ureteric obstruction are often benefited and in many instances cured by removal of the diseased kidney. Removal of a kidney should never be considered lightly, and a trial of medical therapy is always undertaken first. Unilateral nephrectomy is indicated (1) when hypertension is not controlled with medical therapy, (2) if a patient with severe hypertension is noncompliant, or (3) if a patient is unable to tolerate side effects emanating from high doses of antihypertensives required to control his blood pressure.

Severe hypertension in patients with end-stage renal disease (renoprival hypertension) usually responds to dialysis and removal of excess fluid. However, dialysis alone may not be sufficient to control hypertension, and these patients may require additional antihypertensive therapy. Treatment with a combination of furosemide, propranolol, and hydralazine seems to work best in this instance. Minoxidil is an effective vasodilator similar to hydralazine and is probably a better antihypertensive in this situation. The drug will soon be available for clinical use in the United States.

Certain patients with end-stage renal disease requiring chronic maintenance dialysis continue to have severe hypertension despite medical therapy and frequent dialyses. These patients generally have extremely high plasma renin levels. Removal of nonfunctioning kidneys either cures the hypertension or makes it relatively simple to manage with medical therapy.

Renal artery stenosis

If blood pressure is not readily controlled with antihypertensive therapy, surgical treatment is always considered in patients with fibromuscular hyperplasia. A sharply localized single lesion involving the main renal artery in a young patient with a short history of hypertension is ideal for surgical treatment. The revascularization procedures include (1) resection of the stenotic lesion, (2) bypass of the lesion using either a Dacron graft or saphenous vein graft with reestablishment of normal renal blood flow, and (3) endarterectomy with patch plasty. Nephrectomy is considered only if a revascularization procedure is technically impossible or has failed and hypertension cannot be medically controlled.

Fibromuscular hyperplasia is often a bilateral disease and may require bilateral revascularization procedures. Surgical treatment cures hypertension in most of these patients, and in others it increases responsiveness to medical therapy probably by elimination of a renal pressure factor through restoration of normal blood supply to the kidney.

The treatment of choice for patients with atherosclerotic narrowing of the renal artery is medical antihypertensive therapy. Most of these patients have evidence of generalized vascular disease with bilateral renal artery stenosis. They have not only a high operative morbidity but may also die early in the postoperative period of atherosclerotic complications such as myocardial infarction and cerebrovascular accident. Unilateral nephrectomy of an unsalvageable kidney combined with contralateral revascularization is sometimes life-saving and curative of hypertension in certain patients with severe hypertension and extensive atherosclerosis.

Primary aldosteronism

Hypertension in patients with primary aldosteronism due to an aldosterone-secreting adenoma can be controlled with administration of large doses (300 to 400 mg./24 hr.) of spironolactone. Serum potassium concentration also reverses to normal. In the presence of hypertension that is difficult to control, surgery is recommended because of the high rate of cure and certainty of improvement. Resection of the adrenal gland containing the adenoma is the treatment of choice. In one series, 65% of patients with aldosterone-secreting adenoma were cured, and the remainder required much lower dosages of medication for mild hypertension after unilateral adrenalectomy.

Surgical treatment with unilateral or even bilateral adrenalectomy for primary aldosteronism due to bilateral adrenal hyperplasia is unsatisfactory. The effect of spironolactone, 300 to 400 mg./24 hr., on blood pressure in these patients is not as remarkable as in those with an aldosterone-producing adenoma. Additional antihypertensive drugs are generally necessary to control hypertension.

Cushing's syndrome

The treatment of Cushing's syndrome depends on its cause. When the syndrome results from an adrenal tumor, removal of the tumor-bearing gland is curative. Postoperatively, substitute glucocorticoid therapy is essential. Patients with bilateral benign adrenal adenoma require bilateral adrenalectomy followed by lifelong treatment for Addison's disease (adrenal cortical insufficiency). Most patients with adrenal carcinoma have either apparent or occult metastases when first seen. In addition to bilateral adrenalectomy, medical therapy with the adrenocorticolytic drug mitotane (*o,p'*-DDD) induces temporary remission of hyperadrenocorticalism, and in almost 50% of patients, tumor mass regresses for several months to a few years.

When Cushing's syndrome is due to an ectopic ACTH-producing tumor, only in rare instances can it be completely removed. However, with treatment using metyrapone, which inhibits the final step in cortisol synthesis, symptoms of hypercortisolism can be curtailed. Bilateral adrenalectomy or mitotane therapy may be employed in selected patients.

Ideal therapeutic results for Cushing's disease (excessive ACTH production by a pituitary tumor) are achieved by irradiation of the pituitary gland. It is now possible to deliver intensive irradiation to a sharply localized region of the gland with little risk of injuries to neighboring structures. Bilateral adrenalectomy or hypophysectomy are now seldom necessary for treatment of this disorder.

Pheochromocytoma

The treatment of choice is complete surgical excision of the single or multiple tumors. This can be accomplished in almost 90% of patients. Pharmacologic therapy to prevent the physiologic and metabolic effects of catecholamines is effective in reversing the symptoms of the disease in some cases and markedly prolonging life in the remainder. Pharmacologic therapy is also essential before surgery to control the effects of catecholamines.

The α receptor blocking drugs phentolamine (Regitine) and phenoxybenz-amine (Dibenzyline) and the β receptor blocker, propranolol (Inderal), are used for medical treatment of pheochromocytoma. Pharmacology of these drugs has been discussed in Chapter 4. α-Methyl-para-tyrosine is an inhibitor of tyrosine hydroxylase, which is an enzyme necessary for the conversion of tyrosine to dopa. This is a rate-limiting step in the synthesis of catecholamines. The drug is not yet available for clinical use in the United States. It might prove useful in the pharmacologic treatment of pheochromocytoma.

Since there is always a possibility that the patient might have multiple tumors, exploration of the abdomen at the time of surgery is essential. In the immediate postoperative period, many patients develop hypotension requiring fluid and vasopressive therapy. Urine examinations should follow to detect the presence of catecholamine and its metabolites at 6-month intervals to exclude the development of new tumors or metastases.

Coarctation of aorta

The presence of all but mild coarctation requires surgical correction. Some surgeons still prefer to wait until the seventh year before correction; however, recurrence of coarctation after adequate surgical correction has been shown to be negligible.

Resection of coarctation with end-to-end anastomosis or bypass with a Dacron graft are the surgical procedures usually undertaken to correct this condition. Unexplained postoperative hypertension is not uncommon and requires medical therapy.

Toxemia of pregnancy

Since the cause and pathogenesis of toxemia of pregnancy remain undefined, a consensus on its treatment does not exist. Most obstetricians still prefer to treat this condition with intramuscular magnesium sulfate injections and early evacuation of the uterus either by induction of labor or cesarean section. Antihypertensive therapy with diuretics and other pharmacologic agents may help in reversing the hypertension but does not necessarily improve the prognosis for the fetus or mother. Some patients with toxemia have normal or mildly elevated blood pressure but may still succumb to the disease. Hypertension is only one manifestation of an underlying systemic illness, which is almost always reversed after delivery of the fetus.

MANAGEMENT OF HYPERTENSIVE EMERGENCIES

A hypertensive emergency or hypertensive crisis is a clinical situation in which the blood pressure is so elevated as to constitute a threat to life or certain organ systems. Some conditions such as acute left ventricular failure and acute dissecting aneurysm of the aorta qualify as hypertensive emergencies, not so much because of the severity of hypertension but as a result of coexisting life-threatening complications. The clinical situations that constitute hypertensive emergencies can be classified as follows according to the rapidity with which reduction in blood pressure is required:

I. Life-threatening situations requiring immediate reduction in blood pressure
   A. Hypertensive encephalopathy
   B. Acute dissecting aneurysm of the aorta
   C. Acute pulmonary edema (hypertension with acute left ventricular failure)
II. Situations requiring urgent reduction in blood pressure
   A. Malignant or accelerated hypertension
   B. Intracerebral or subarachnoid hemorrhage
   C. Severe hypertension in a patient with acute coronary insufficiency or myocardial infarction
III. Situations requiring relatively rapid reduction in blood pressure
   A. Diastolic blood pressure above 130 mm. Hg
   B. Hypertension associated with acute glomerulonephritis
IV. Curable conditions that may require prompt reduction in blood pressure
   A. Pheochromocytoma
   B. Toxemia of pregnancy
   C. Oral contraceptive–induced severe hypertension
   D. Renovascular hypertension

Management of hypertensive emergencies usually requires intravenous administration of antihypertensive drugs. The medications presently used include furosemide (Lasix), sodium nitroprusside (Nipride), diazoxide (Hyperstat), and trimethaphan (Arfonad). The clinical pharmacology of these drugs has been described in Chapter 4.

During administration of these potent antihypertensive agents, close monitoring of arterial blood pressure, preferably using an interarterial line, is essential, and these patients are therefore best treated in an intensive care setting.

Clinical features and the management of some hypertensive emergencies are discussed in the following sections.

Hypertensive encephalopathy

Hypertensive encephalopathy is characterized by severe headache, nausea, vomiting, visual blurring or blindness, and transient neurologic disturbances including local and generalized seizures. The fundi show grade iii or iv hypertensive changes, and the blood pressure is usually above 250/150 mm. Hg. The syndrome may complicate acute glomerulonephritis, toxemia of pregnancy, and malignant hypertension. The clinical manifestations are probably secondary to cerebral edema. With increasing use of diuretics in the management of essential hypertension, the syndrome of hypertensive encephalopathy has become uncommon during the past ten years.

Differentiation of hypertensive encephalopathy from acute cerebrovascular accident is frequently necessary. The second condition is almost always associated with localizing neurologic signs that do not improve with reduction in blood pressure.

The condition requires immediate reduction in blood pressure. We prefer to use intravenous furosemide in a bolus form and sodium nitroprusside infusion to titrate the blood pressure. The aim is to maintain diastolic blood pressure at about 100 to 110 mm. Hg by regulating the dose of sodium nitroprusside. Furosemide injection (40 to 80 mg.) is repeated every 4 to 6 hours to maintain urine flow.

Reserpine is best avoided in this situation because it alters the level of consciousness, which needs to be monitored for continuing evaluation of patient's condition.

Acute dissecting aneurysm of aorta

In an acute dissecting aneurysm of aorta, a tear occurs in the wall of the ascending or the arch of the aorta through which blood enters the wall of the aorta, splits the media of the vessel, and enters the lumen through another tear distally, forming a dissecting hematoma. Congenital diseases such as medial cystic necrosis and Marfan's syndrome predispose to dissection of the aorta. The relation of hypertension to a dissecting aneurysm is not clear and atheromatous disease of the aorta does not result in medial cystic necrosis. Dissecting aneurysm of the aorta is far less common than myocardial infarction but is a more serious disorder. The peak incidence is in the fourth to seventh decades of life.

Dissecting aneurysm is frequently confused with myocardial infarction, pulmonary embolism, acute abdominal crisis, or peripheral vascular occlusions. The patient usually experiences severe anterior chest pain radiating to the back. Blood pressure is elevated in most patients, although they may appear to be in a shocklike state. Absence or inequality of carotid, brachial, radial, and femoral pulsations is an important clue in indicating arterial occlusion. The early diastolic murmur of aortic regurgitation may be heard in about one third of patients. Neurologic abnormalities are common and result from occlusion of the brain or spinal cord arteries. Some patients complain of abdominal pain because of ischemia of the visceral organs. Involvement of renal arteries may cause hematuria, oliguria, and aggravation of hypertension. Chest x-ray examination shows widening of the aorta. Aortogram is necessary for definitive diagnosis and shows a double lumen.

Until recently dissecting aneurysm of the aorta was considered a surgical disease and had a mortality from 50% to 100% even in the best hands. Now it is considered a medical illness. Pain is relieved with the use of morphine. Antihypertensive therapy is initiated with intravenous furosemide and trimethaphan. Systolic blood pressure should be reduced to 100 to 120 mm. Hg. It is maintained at that level with the use of intramuscular reserpine and oral guanethidine. Furosemide is repeated as indicated to maintain urine flow. Surgery is only indicated when the patient has overwhelming aortic valve insufficiency, drug therapy fails to halt progression of the dissecting hematoma, blood starts to leak from the aneurysm, or a major branch of the aorta is occluded.

Acute pulmonary edema

Acute left ventricular failure may be precipitated by severe hypertension with or without myocardial infarction. The common signs of pulmonary edema such as acute shortness of breath, cyanosis, gallop rhythm, and pulsus alternans are present. Most patients respond satisfactorily to the standard treatment measures, consisting of intravenous furosemide, digitalis, morphine, oxygen, and use of rotating tourniquets. When these measures fail, a more direct attack on the elevated arterial pressure using intravenous sodium nitroprusside is recommended even when the blood pressure is not excessively high.

Malignant or accelerated hypertension

The difference between malignant and accelerated hypertension is quantitative rather than qualitative. The condition is labeled "malignant hypertension" when the diastolic blood pressure is above 150 mm. Hg and the fundi show papilledema. It is termed "accelerated hypertension" when the fundi show grade iii changes (hemorrhages and exudates without papilledema) and the diastolic blood pressure is above 130 mm. Hg.

In most tissues the arterioles demonstrate fibrinoid necrosis where the vessel wall is replaced by eosinophilic granular material with loss of cell nuclei and reduction of the lumen. Occasionally polymorphonuclear and mononuclear cells may be present, a pathologic picture for which the term "necrotizing arteriolitis" is used.

Aggressive antihypertensive treatment improves survival. The aim of the therapy is to keep the diastolic blood pressure below 110 mm. Hg. Therapy should be instituted first and investigations for secondary hypertension performed later. Intravenous furosemide and diazoxide are the treatment of choice. Oral antihypertensive medications such as methyldopa and a diuretic are started simultaneously so that the blood pressure can be maintained at a lower level without the need of parenteral antihypertensive drugs.

Failure to control blood pressure eventually results in renal failure. In many patients, lowering of blood pressure may lead to transient elevation in BUN and creatinine levels, but the long-term survival rate is definitely improved with therapy.

Intracerebral or subarachnoid hemorrhage

Intracerebral or subarachnoid hemorrhage is a hypertensive crisis that occurs more often in blacks than in whites. The diastolic blood pressure is usually above 120 mm. Hg. The fundi show grade ii or iii hypertensive changes. The level of consciousness is altered. If the patient is conscious, occipital headache is usually the major complaint. Nuchal rigidity and lateralizing signs are almost always present.

The aim of therapy is to reduce diastolic blood pressure to a level of 100 to 110 mm. Hg. Intravenous furosemide and diazoxide are usually the antihypertensive agents of choice. Simultaneous oral therapy with a diuretic and methyldopa or propranolol can be started to keep hypertension under control. Reserpine and clonidine, which cause drowsiness and complicate the clinical picture, should be avoided.

Acute coronary insufficiency

Persistent ischemic cardiac pain is usually a forewarning of impending myocardial infarction. Severe hypertension in this setting generally follows rather than precedes the onset of coronary insufficiency. Extreme anxiety and myocardial ischemia may produce a reflex increase in blood pressure. The extremely elevated blood pressure further embarrasses an ischemic left ventricular muscle making the condition worse.

The aim of treatment is to reduce blood pressure to a moderate level such as 100 mm. Hg diastolic. Intramuscular reserpine, which brings about a fall in blood pressure in 2 to 4 hours and produces sedation, is probably the drug of choice. Treatment is continued with oral diuretics and reserpine.

Severe hypertension

Patients who have diastolic blood pressure equal to or above 120 mm. Hg are considered to have severe hypertension and require relatively rapid reduction in blood pressure. If the patient is asymptomatic, chances are that he has had hypertension for several weeks if not months or years. In the absence of a hypertensive crisis situation, it is usually not necessary to admit such patients to hospital. Outpatient treatment with a diuretic along with a step II drug (methyldopa, propranolol, prazosin, clonidine, or reserpine) usually brings the blood pressure down to a safe level.

If the diastolic blood pressure is 130 mm. Hg or above, even in the absence of symptoms, hospitalization with bed rest is probably indicated because such patients are in danger of developing malignant hypertension, hypertension encephalopathy, or one of the other crisis situations.

When a patient with suspected secondary hypertension presents with severe hypertension or is in a hypertensive crisis, prompt reduction of blood pressure is the first aim of therapy. After the blood pressure has been reasonably controlled, appropriate investigations can be performed for a specific diagnosis.

In summary, the nurse's role in hypertensive emergencies is early identification, immediate medical referral, initiation of prescribed therapy, monitoring clinical parameters, providing patient/family support and explanation, and the coordination of services.

A crisis of reluctance?

Although hypertensive crises have diminished in frequency in the past decade, the primary crisis is the reluctance to treat and follow up patients with mild to moderate hypertension. The best way to manage hypertensive and atherosclerotic emergencies is to prevent them by early detection and treatment of hypertension. Even if a physician elects to defer treatment of mild hypertension, the patient must have his blood pressure checked regularly. In the event of further elevations, appropriate antihypertensive therapy can be instituted without delay.

SUMMARY

Nurse-managed hypertension clinics are proving successful. This chapter provides the nurse with detailed information on actual management of hypertension.

Behavioral methods such as biofeedback, relaxation techniques, psychotherapy, suggestion, and environmental modification are becoming increasingly popular as adjunctive measures in treatment of hypertension.

Antihypertensive medications are the mainstay of treatment of hypertension. In stepped-care therapy of essential hypertension, the treatment is initiated with a diuretic and other antihypertensives are added as necessary. Pretreatment considerations include knowledge of the patient's allergies, contraindications to certain drugs, and potential drug interactions. Detailed pretreatment counseling is helpful. It is useful to classify the hypertensive as labile, mild, moderate, or severe, depending on the level of the blood pressure for appropriate therapy. The patient should be monitored for compliance, blood pressure control, symptoms, and side effects at appropriate intervals. Side effects common to many antihypertensives are dry mouth, lethargy, dizziness, sexual dysfunction, and weight gain. Complications or adverse effects vary from one drug to the other.

Treatment of secondary hypertension depends on the cause. A trial of medical therapy is indicated in certain instances. In some cases, surgical treatment can cure the hypertension. Even if a cure is not achieved after surgery, it is much easier to control blood pressure medically in many patients.

Hypertensive emergencies are clinical situations in which hypertension constitutes a threat to life and certain organ systems. Their management usually requires intravenous administration of antihypertensive drugs. Furosemide, sodium nitroprusside, diazoxide, and trimethaphen are some of the drugs indicated in the treatment of hypertensive emergencies.

The incidence of hypertensive crises has greatly diminished in the past decade. The reluctance to treat and follow up patients with mild to moderate hypertension may be the important crisis of today.

SUGGESTED READINGS

1. Report of the Joint National Committee on Detection, Evaluation, and Treatment of High Blood Pressure, J.A.M.A. **237:**255-261, 1977.
2. Shapiro, A. G., Schwartz, G. E., Ferguson, D. C. E., Redmond, D. P., and Weiss, S. M.: Behavioral methods in the treatment of hypertension, Ann. Intern. Med. **86:**626-636, 1977.

CHAPTER 6

Counseling the hypertensive

All health care delivery workers participate in the educational process involved in the maintenance or restoration of health; however, the nurse's role is strategic. Patients and families can be assisted in learning health principles and practices if every opportunity and appropriate setting are utilized for teaching purposes. They can be guided toward assuming responsibility for applying or incorporating that new knowledge.

Hypertension control services are provided in a variety of settings: hospitals, clinics, private practice offices, homes, schools, and industrial and business establishments. Although nurses may be well equipped with principles and strategies for the teaching/learning process, it is necessary to formulate a personal philosophy and commitment toward patient education and hypertension control. This will initiate the operational framework and objectives for patient education in each unique nursing care setting.

OVERVIEW OF COUNSELING PROCESS

The development of an education component in hypertension control is predicated on the humanistic consideration that all hypertensive or potentially hypertensive individuals must be provided the necessary information to act in their own best interest. During the blood pressure screening process, or phase 1, the nurse's ability to impart the necessary information regarding high blood pressure, thereby alerting the patient to acquire medical care, is crucial. With this frame of reference the patient enters the health care system and begins to participate in a therapeutic relationship with the involved professionals. Hence a thorough understanding of the concept of hypertension, related factors, patient needs and abilities, and various teaching strategies is required. We have endeavored to

85

provide the highlights of the counseling process as performed in their clinical setting. Brief simple patient explanations are presented for ease of adaptability and expansion of content to address individual patient and family needs.

PHASE I: COUNSELING THROUGH THE BLOOD PRESSURE SCREENING PROCESS

At the initial blood pressure screening session, health care workers performing the blood pressure reading must obtain identifying information. During that series of questions, the attitude, tone, interest, and warmth conveyed by the health care worker sets the interactional framework.

A brief, simple explanation defining blood pressure is usually the starting place. Depending on the client's ability, the basic definition can be as follows:

Blood pressure is the force of blood pressing against the blood vessel wall. The heart is the muscle pumping the blood through the body. When the heart is squeezing or pumping, there is a greater pressure or force pushing the blood through the blood vessel. This is called "systolic blood pressure," or the top number in the blood pressure reading. When the heart is resting between beats, there is less pressure in the blood vessel. This is called "diastolic blood pressure," or the bottom number in the blood pressure reading. In some people, the blood pressure goes up and stays up most of the time. This is called "high blood pressure," or "hypertension." Hypertension then is continuous or sustained high blood pressure.

The procedure for blood pressure measurement can also be described. Common misconceptions such as pain or the use of needles can thus be promptly dispelled. Eliciting client questions at this time assists the health care worker in assessing that individual's learning abilities and promotes their interaction.

The next major focus of the counseling process is directed at the prevalence and risk of hypertension, its silent but deadly nature, and the need for medical management. Depending on the individual or general clientele involved, the following points are the most relevant and meaningful to stress during counseling:

1. Approximately 50 million Americans have high blood pressure. Almost 50% of these may not know they have the condition, and many who do know are not under a physician's treatment.
2. More men have hypertension than women.
3. More blacks have hypertension than whites.
4. Individuals with a family history of high blood pressure, heart or kidney problems, stroke, or diabetes may have a greater chance for having high blood pressure. Getting yearly blood pressure checks is a family affair.
5. The children of parents with high blood pressure are more prone to develop hypertension. Even slightly higher blood pressure readings in young persons can mean serious later complications.
6. The higher the blood pressure level the more serious the risk of early death and complications such as heart failure, stroke, or kidney disease.

7. Smoking by an individual with high blood pressure causes more heart damage.
8. Hypertension is a silent disease; there are no characteristic or certain set of symptoms. Symptoms such as headache, dizziness, shortness of breath, flushing, and tingling may be from high blood pressure; these may also be caused by other health problems. Therefore a physician's evaluation is necessary and strongly advised. These symptoms may be warning signs before a major problem occurs.
9. Since the damage from hypertension occurs slowly and continuously, especially if not treated, long-term physician's care is absolutely necessary. This means it is important to get under a physician's care and continue with it.
10. The medical profession does not know the exact cause for hypertension, but high blood pressure can be controlled.

With an elevated blood pressure reading, the client is informed of our referral criteria. The necessity of returning for a second blood pressure check and/or obtaining further medical evaluation should be emphatically communicated to the client. Strategies that may be employed to motivate these individuals include giving informational pamphlets, utilizing family support, prompt scheduling for the second blood pressure check with not more than a week's lapse in time, and imparting a genuine personal concern. Additional motivational principles and strategies are discussed in Chapter 7. Follow-up of these individuals is absolutely necessary to ensure that they have indeed acquired medical care.

PHASE II: COUNSELING HYPERTENSIVE PATIENTS IN A HEALTH CARE SETTING

The suspected hypertensive who has now entered the health care system for the treatment of hypertension presents an exciting challenge to the nurse during the initial visits. Assuming the patient has had no previous benefits of hypertension counseling, the nurse may embark on the counseling format as previously described. The difference is that a more extensive assessment of learning abilities and readiness and the consideration of psychosocial adaptation to a long-term illness are necessary. Within our experience, initially incorporating counseling approaches during the health history performed by the nurse has been most successful.

The well-known principles of learning that are the basis for a hypertension patient education program include the following[9,10]:

- Motivation as the key factor
- Immediate meaningful feedback
- Positive reinforcement as an incentive
- Teaching interventions that are meaningful, organized, and relevant and elicit active learner participation
- Teaching strategies that are varied and individualized, with intermittent reinforcement to remotivate

Detailed applications of these principles are incorporated throughout the text.

Assessment of learning abilities and readiness

Patient perceptions, priorities, and needs; factors that may enhance or block learning; and their current knowledge of hypertension and its meaning to them can be assessed with a series of pertinent questions. This may include the following:

1. *Patient perceptions, priorities, and motivations.* What reason does the patient define for acquiring medical care at this time? What are the precipitating circumstances and motivations directing the patient's actions? How does the patient accept the need for obtaining medical evaluation? How has stress or anxiety influenced the patient's coping and perceptual abilities? What does the patient and family define as their priorities and needs?

2. *Factors that may enhance or block the learning process.* Does the patient have the physical and mental readiness necessary for learning? In terms of ability to communicate, what are the patient's strengths and weaknesses? Are there any errors in the patient's perceptions about the current situation? Will the patient's priorities and motivations be receptive to learning? Will the family participate in and support the medical care? Which teaching strategies will best suit the patient?

3. *Level of intelligence.* What level of formal education has the patient completed? Can the patient read and write? Does the attention span appear short?

4. *Current knowledge of hypertension.* What was the patient and family's previous experience with hypertension and what does hypertension currently mean to them?

Teaching strategies

Once the assessment has been completed, full attention can be directed at extensive counseling. Initially a one-to-one teaching strategy is employed. During the course of clinic visits, the four teaching strategies of the one-to-one approach, written materials, audiovisual presentations, and the group process are continuously utilized. Accommodations need to be made as to which teaching strategy best addresses current patient needs. Blanket teaching interventions for groups of patients are not helpful. If individuals have basic needs or urgent priorities that are unmet, interventions aimed at learning alone are not appropriate.

The goal of the *one-to-one* teaching strategy is to personally provide the patient and family with the basic highlights of hypertension counseling. In addition, the opportunity for the patient to specifically question and problem solve is an inherent component of this approach. In patients whose learning abilities are marginal, this method has proved most successful in our setting. This strategy is incorporated into the nurse's interview at each clinic visit and is documented.

The goal of using *written materials* is to clarify and reinforce one-to-one counseling. In addition, these ready references can be utilized by other family members to enlist the necessary support. Initially the patient is provided with the clinic orientation pamphlet, which is followed by the patient hypertension handbook that we have developed, and other appropriate pamphlets. These are reviewed at each clinic visit as necessary. We use materials that are written at various levels of difficulty, directed at individual learning abilities and readiness. For example, we distribute extremely simple, profusely illustrated material to patients who have reading difficulties. For these patients, we employ the one-to-one approach, audiovisual aids, and group process more extensively.

Patients who exhibit strong denial or obstinance or refuse to participate in or accept counseling are given a few concisely and simply written materials of a more personalized quality. Audiovisual and group process approaches seem to be more helpful in these situations.

On the other hand, compliant patients who have progressed through and assimilated the basic information are given more comprehensive, detailed materials.

The *audiovisual presentations* are 6- to 10-minute slide or film sessions conducted with groups of patients. The content varies and initially consists of the basic understanding of hypertension, diet, and medication therapy. The question-and-answer sessions preceding and following the program are particularly enlightening. The goal of this strategy is to more vividly communicate the essence of the nature of hypertension and its treatment. The analogues presented in the films and slides aid the patient's understanding by comparing various aspects of hypertension to commonly understood concepts and processes. Charts and diagrams further focus the patient.

The *group sessions* effectively assist the patient and family through peer support of common concerns and questions. The goal of this strategy is to utilize the group environment to be as conducive as possible to peer and staff interaction, further enhancing the patient's understanding. This strategy is employed at each clinic visit and documented.

Thus the manner in which these strategies are utilized depends on patient and family needs and the availability of resources and personnel.

Prior to the newly diagnosed hypertensive and family participating in a counseling program, consideration must be given to their *psychosocial adaptation*. The stages of adaptation are categorized as follows: shock and disbelief, increasing awareness, reorganization, resolution, and assumption of a new identity.

Initially, during the shock and disbelief phase, patients and their families feel overwhelmed and anxious. They do not hear much of what they are told. They focus on one or two words or ideas during the interaction. Consequently the words and approaches employed by the clinician at this point are crucial. Imparting only the essential information in a well-focused manner is necessary. The nature of hypertension, progression, complications, and chronic nature can be addressed. Details and goals of treatment can be discussed only in terms of the alternatives available, since additional information may be confusing. Taking prescribed medications is considered the easiest health behavior to adapt to, since it is additive and does not change life-style dramatically. Patients and their families need to be oriented to clinic services and procedures and what to expect in the initial and subsequent visits. Nurses can convey warmth, concern, and their availability to discuss patients' feelings, illness, and questions or problems.

If a patient fails to appear at the subsequent appointment, personalized outreach procedures can be instituted. Listening with empathy is crucial at this time. If the patient appears overanxious, attempt to discuss these feelings and determine their cause prior to initiating counseling.

During the second stage patients and their families become increasingly aware of the disease, its personal meaning, and its implications and threat. Many questions are raised and must be answered honestly and on an individualized basis. The rapport established earlier with the nurse facilitates the development of trust in this phase. Patients and their families are now more likely to participate in a hypertension education program, and the interest level is higher.

The third phase, reorganization, involves the recognition by patients of their hypertension. They are more flexible in terms of adapting and adjusting to the therapeutic regimen. Positive steps are now made to incorporate the therapy and life-style changes into their daily patterns of living and working. Clarification and reinforcement of teaching aspects can be easily done. Patients are more able to objectively evaluate their progress in terms of the hypertension, treatment, and life-style changes.

During the last stages, resolution and assumption of a new identity, patients have fully incorporated the therapeutic regimen into their daily life. They readily acknowledge that they are hypertensive.

In the clinical spectrum, patients and their families progress through various stages of this process again and again. Furthermore, many individuals never reach the final stage.

Counseling aspects

In addition to the counseling aspects stressed during the blood pressure screening procedure, other considerations may now be emphasized. The nurse can begin by explaining that the cause of hypertension is not known at this time:

> Over 95% of individuals who have high blood pressure have the essential type of hypertension. The other 5% have secondary hypertension, the causes of which are usually known, such as kidney problems.

Certain conditions or factors may make an individual more prone to develop hypertension. These are called "predisposing factors." During counseling, these predisposing factors can be identified, evaluated, and modified as jointly negotiated.

Heredity. As the patient's family history is explored, particular attention should be directed at cardiovascular, cerebrovascular, renal, and diabetic conditions. If one or more of these conditions are present, the counselor should stress the increased chances of having high blood pressure with various target organ complications. In addition, the chances of having high blood pressure are approximately two times greater if either a parent or brother or sister have high blood pressure, so getting yearly blood pressure checks are a family affair.

Individuals may inherit a propensity for hypertension that can be manifested if they are exposed to certain environmental conditions such as stress, obesity, and a high-salt diet. Therefore an individual with a positive family history of high blood pressure who has any of the contributory environmental factors present is in greater danger for developing high blood pressure. Simply stated, certain conditions such as being overweight, eating too much salt, and having stressful problems can cause high blood pressure to appear sooner and more severely.

Involving family members in the counseling sessions aids in enlisting their understanding and participation in the care of that family member. Furthermore, modification of environmental contributory factors is a family effort at preventive health care.

Race. When counseling black patients, race as a special component of heredity can be discussed. Generally, hypertension is more common among black than white individuals. There are theories as to the reason for this serious problem, but none have been proved. High-salt intake in "soul food" and the anxiety and stress generated by inner-city living conditions have been weighed heavily.

Smoking. Smoking presents a common and particularly frustrating area in patient education. Despite all the publicity and efforts at consumer education about the dangers of smoking, cigarette sales have increased in the past few years! Furthermore, when people decrease smoking, the dietary intake may increase. This phenomena is well recognized and has been statistically documented in our setting.

Smoking is an independent risk factor in that alone it is not a cause of hypertension, but smoking by an individual with a hypertensive propensity or condition can contribute to more serious complications. Available data have demonstrated that young men entering college with a systolic pressure of 130 mm. Hg or above and smoking ten or more cigarettes a day incurred a 110% increase in the risk of coronary death.[12]

The physiologic effects of smoking include increased heart rate, peripheral vasoconstriction, damage to the ciliary lining of the bronchioles, and altered oxygen concentrations in the respiratory system and blood. Furthermore, effects of nicotine and/or carbon monoxide on the processes involving free fatty acids and platelets have been documented. However, atherosclerosis does not seem to be directly affected. The continuous strain that smoking, hypercholestremia, and high blood pressure place on the coronary circulation are additive and deadly.

The risks to the cigar smoking population is not considerable, since these individuals usually do not inhale.

Dividing the patient population into the following four categories assists with the assessment and determination of appropriate counseling strategies:

1. None or occasional cigarette or cigar smoking
2. Less than one pack a day
3. One to two packs a day
4. More than two packs a day

All patients must be counseled regarding the physiologic effects of smoking, the added risks of smoking with high blood pressure, and the increased chances of coronary heart disease, lung cancer, and emphysema.

Patients who smoke less than one pack of cigarettes a day (category 2) require more assistance than general counseling. The nurse can promote self-evaluation on the part of these patients by exploring the reasons for their smoking practices. Suggestions may include writing a personal card citing the reasons for the smoking practices. Keeping a daily table briefly describing the circumstances surrounding the smoking experience and the number of cigarettes smoked may be helpful. After a week, repetitive patterns that lead to expectations and cravings begin to emerge. Posing new questions such as, "Do I really need this cigarette or is this a reflex?" aids the introspective process. Exploring which stresses in particular elicit frequent strong smoking experiences is also helpful.

With this insight and understanding, the nurse and patient can jointly explore acceptable methods of decreasing smoking practices with the goal of eventual elimination. Following is a possible approach to patient explanation:

> Don't smoke, if possible. Smoking makes the heart beat faster, raises blood pressure, upsets the flow of air and blood in your lungs, and damages the lining in your lungs. The constant strain that smoking, high-fat diet, and high blood pressure places on the heart add up and are deadly. Some ways to begin "kicking the habit" are:
>
> 1. Choose a cigarette with less tar and nicotine.
> 2. Smoke only the first half of the cigarette.
> 3. Reduce the number of times a puff is taken on a cigarette.
> 4. Reduce the depth of inhalation.
> 5. Smoke fewer cigarettes a day.
> 6. Exercise more.
> 7. Pursue new hobbies and interests.
> 8. Find a safe substitute for handling cigarettes like a lucky coin, pen, or pencil.
>
> Sometimes people who are trying to quit smoking begin to gain weight. Keeping low calorie foods and beverages within easy reach helps, instead of a cigarette.

The list of tips to stop smoking are endless and challenge the creative ability of the nurse to adapt and personalize the patient's management.

Patients who smoke an excess of a pack a day (categories 3 and 4) are exceedingly more difficult to motivate. Stronger encouragement, guidance, and support are required. Any variety of approaches may be utilized, depending on the patient's needs, desire to quit smoking, and abilities. Antismoking group sessions may prove to be of added value with these particular individuals.

Birth control pills and pregnancy. The incidence of hypertension in women who take birth control pills is twice that of women who do not. Of women who take oral contraceptives 5% to 7% develop hypertension as a side effect. Normotensive women with a positive family history for high blood pressure and cardiac, renal, cerebrovascular, or diabetic conditions are at risk for developing hypertension and should avoid birth control pills.

Routinely, all women taking oral contraceptives need a blood pressure measurement at least every 6 months. If hypertension develops, the advice is to discontinue the pills. Alternate forms of birth control should promptly be instituted, and frequent observation is required with possible pharmacologic therapy until the blood pressure levels have normalized.

If birth control pills must be continued or if estrogen must be given for other indications, the blood pressure needs to be checked monthly or more frequently and antihypertensive drug therapy initiated. Close observation is necessary to ensure adequate blood pressure control.

Pregnancy-induced hypertension, or preeclampsia, is a significant problem. Women with hypertensive cardiovascular disease prior to pregnancy are at considerable risk for developing preeclampsia. Any pregnant woman with a blood pressure greater than 125/85 mm. Hg or an increase greater than 30 mm. Hg systolic and/or 15 mm. Hg diastolic requires close obstetric observation.

A moderate to severely hypertensive woman needs to seriously consider avoiding pregnancy may be so advised. This is because many obstetricians will discontinue the antihypertensive medication to prevent fetal damage and avoid altered fluid and electrolyte levels. If the patient becomes pregnant, it is imperative that an obstetrician be involved immediately.

Thus the medical emphasis is as follows:

1. Do not prescribe birth control pills to hypertensive women or those at risk for developing hypertension.
2. Discontinue birth control pills if hypertension develops.
3. If moderately or severely hypertensive, the woman should avoid pregnancy.
4. If she does become pregnant, close obstetric observation and management are necessary to prevent preeclampsia.

The patient explanation may be as follows:

Women who take birth control pills double their chances of having high blood pressure. The exact reason is not known yet, but physicians do know that the hormones in the pills cause your body to hold in more salt and water, which could raise your blood pressure. Be sure to tell your physician if you or your family have high blood pressure, heart or kidney problems, stroke, or diabetes.

This may mean your chances of having hypertension are greater, and perhaps another type of birth control may be better, depending on the doctor's evaluation and advice.

If you are taking birth control pills or hormones for change of life, you need to see your physician regularly and have your blood pressure checked at least every 6 months. If your blood pressure does become high, your physician will decide what is best. The physician may stop the pill and prescribe different birth control ways or continue to prescribe the pill or hormones, as well as other medicines. In that case, your blood pressure will be checked more often.

Many women ask, "Can I have high blood pressure if I am pregnant?" The answer is "Yes, pregnant women can develop high blood pressure." This condition is called "preeclampsia," or "toxemia." The exact cause is not known, but physicians do know that if you had high blood pressure before you were pregnant, your chances for having high blood pressure complications during pregnancy is higher. You will need to visit the doctor more often and follow his advice closely.

The danger signs, which can alert the pregnant woman to see the physician are headaches, vision problems, puffy eyelids, swelling of hands, ankles, and feet, and more of a weight gain than the doctor advises. After the baby is born, the high blood pressure usually returns to the levels before pregnancy. But these women still have a better chance for having hypertension as time goes on.

Alcohol. Alcohol consumption is assessed during the history interview. Precise, sensitive questioning may be necessary to elicit an accurate amount of daily intake. Frequently, patients are reluctant, embarrassed, or ashamed to state the amounts actually consumed. We categorize alcohol intake in the following manner:

1. None or occasional
2. Alcohol consumption confined to weekends
3. Alcohol consumption totaling no more than 2 drinks a day
4. Alcohol consumption totaling more than 2 drinks a day

We consider that many patients in category 4 are probably alcoholics requiring care of this disease.

It is worthy to note what types of liquor an individual prefers. Certainly the clinical implications of consuming a quart of beer differ from that of consuming a quart of wine or vodka a day because of the variation in the percentage and strength of alcohol content.

The Framingham study documents a modest but definite effect of alcohol on high blood pressure.[3,4] According to their results, the first drink lowers blood pressure. However, as the patient consumes more, the blood pressure rises. Once beyond the moderate intake range, the blood pressure progressively elevates. The Kaiser-Permanente study verifies this and further demonstrates that three or more drinks daily is a definite risk factor for hypertension.[6]

Alcohol consumption on weekends, particularly in the adolescent and young adult population, often dramatically increases. This habit may persist later in life. The clinical significance of this practice is that the fluid challenge imposed on the cardiovascular system may, in the presence of mild renal insufficiency and a relatively rigid vascular system with atherosclerosis, produce temporary but severe elevations in blood pressure.

Heavy alcohol consumption may damage the myocardium with consequent cardiomyopathy. In the presence of hypertension and atherosclerosis, even mild cardiomyopathy can produce serious disability. Consequently, hypertensive individuals should be counseled to reduce their alcohol consumption.

An accurate assessment of previous and current alcohol consumption is needed. Questions such as "How many drinks do you have per day?" and "How many shots of alcohol are in one drink?" may be helpful. For further assessment of weekend drinking, questions may be phrased in the following manner: "How many six-packs of beer do you drink in a weekend?" or "How many pints of vodka do you drink over the weekend?" If the patient drinks with companions and shares the bottle, questions such as "How many friends do you share the bottle with and how many bottles are used?" are helpful. More specific questioning is usually needed to determine more exact amounts and frequency of consumption with category 2, 3, and 4 individuals.

The nurse can then proceed to explain the effects and consequences of alcohol consumption. Additional risks to the circulatory system with hypertension may be defined. All patients are in need of the benefits of counseling regardless of the actual alcohol intake. The preventive aspects with the nondrinking population require emphasis.

Individuals whose alcohol intake places them in a moderate to heavy range (categories 2 to 4) require further guidance and extensive family support. The patient's needs and motivations for the alcohol consumptions patterns can be jointly explored with the nurse. The family's participation is crucial. Promoting the introspective process and encouraging insight with support is a sensitive and difficult process. With this basis, the nurse can better assist the patient and family to find the appropriate methods and resources for decreasing the alcohol intake.

Following is a possible brief patient explanation:

> Drinking alcohol is a risk with high blood pressure. Although the first drink may lower blood pressure a little, the blood pressure will rise with more alcohol. Heavy weekend drinking may be a real problem. Large amounts of alcohol, especially over a short period of time with high blood pressure, place a tremendous strain on the heart and circulation. Also, alcohol and high blood pressure medications can sometimes be a dangerous combination. So, take your medicine daily and limit your drinking.
> 1. Try low calorie beer.
> 2. Limit the number and kind of drinks; in other words, have less drinks and avoid strong liquors.
> 3. Buy smaller amounts.
> 4. Drink other beverages like soda, milk, coffee, tea, or fruit juice.

Physician collaboration is essential for medical evaluation of the physiologic and psychiatric consequences of this illness. Numerous community and religious agencies are directed at the alcoholic and his family and can be utilized.

Exercise. The question of what exercise and physical conditioning can do for blood pressure is controversial.[5] It is known that during exercise the systolic pressure increases and the diastolic pressure decreases in a normal individual.

A sedentary individual who is not in good physical condition can have a different response; the diastolic pressure rises during exercise, thereby creating a potentially dangerous situation. Myocardial infarction and cerebrovascular accidents are well documented in these particular individuals who suddenly undertake heavy snow shoveling or moving heavy objects.

In terms of the relationship between exercise and cardiovascular disease, the Framingham study found that individuals who are more physically active have lower rates of cardiovascular disease. However, the relationship between exercise and hypertension has not been studied to a significant degree.

Medical authorities unanimously agree that individuals with cardiovascular disease, severe hypertension, or both should be evaluated by their physician prior to undertaking an exercise or physical conditioning program. This evaluation may include monitoring blood pressure while exercising in a controlled situation such as on a treadmill.

If the physician approves an exercise or physical conditioning program, a gradually accelerated course is advised. Two types of exercise can be discussed. Isotonic exercise is active muscle movement involving a change in the muscle length with minimal tension difference. This includes swimming, bicycling, running, and rhythmic calisthenics. This dynamic muscle activity requires additional oxygen consumption with a subsequent increase in cardiac and respiratory rate and volume. However, the blood pressure does not dramatically change.

Isometric exercise or passive muscle activity increases muscle tension. There is minimal change in the length of the muscles. This includes lifting heavy objects or pressing weights. The heart rate increases slightly, but a significant rise in blood pressure occurs. The neurologic reflexes arising from these tense muscles mediate vasoconstriction and increase the pumping action of the heart with a rapid and considerable elevation in blood pressure.

For the hypertensive patient, daily isotonic exercise can be encouraged and isometric exercise discouraged. Advice such as more walking and proper body mechanics for lifting or moving objects is helpful.

The type of antihypertensive medication prescribed merits additional consideration. Sympathetic inhibitor drugs such as guanethidine (Ismelin) can precipitate profound hypotensive effects during exercise or rapid position changes. Caution is advised when patients are receiving this drug.

A patient explanation may be as follows:

> Everyone should do some type of exercise daily. If you have hypertension or any other disease, you need your physician's advice before starting an exercise

program. Usually a slowly advanced approach to exercising is advised. An example may be to walk two blocks a day and slowly add on more blocks and speed until you are jogging a mile a day. But this depends on your physician's orders. Generally, exercises like running, walking, swimming, and bicycling lower your blood pressure and are very good. These are called "isotonic" types of exercise. But exercises like pressing weights or lifting heavy objects can cause a very fast and high blood pressure change. These are called "isometric" types of exercises and should be avoided.

Lengthier and more detailed explanations can accompany a prescription exercise program.

The effects of drug therapy on position changes and patient counseling is discussed in Chapter 5.

Stress and relaxation. The possible etiologic and catalytic relationships of stress to hypertension are now being studied more extensively. The physiologic responses that prepare the individual for fight or flight are clearly documented.

Although human physiologic responses to threat are uniform, there are rapid, complex psychologic alterations that are integrated with the physiologic responses. Dr. Herbert Benson[1] purports that the continuous behavioral alterations necessitated by stressful environmental conditions may be translated in the central nervous system into the hemodynamic processes that may evolve into essential hypertension.

How humans can alter and learn to control their physiologic responses to stress is a controversial area. The basis for this was originally investigated by B. F. Skinner,[11] his premise being that if one manipulates the environment, behavior could be controlled.

Later Dr. Neil Miller's studies[8] demonstrated that involuntary behavior regulated by the autonomic nervous system could be changed by the biofeedback process. It is believed that through this process of visceral learning, the person recognizes a biologic event, thereby acquiring control of it. This was demonstrated in studies on blood flow in an animal's ear, heart rate, and blood pressure.

In the 1960s transcendental meditation (TM) came into vogue as a way to escape stress and environmental pressures without the use of chemicals or drugs. Through this altered state of consciousness, individuals felt increased energy, well-being, and lowered stress levels. Dr. Benson and others at Harvard University investigated the physiologic changes that occurred during TM. Their findings revealed that there were definite physiologic responses which accompanied meditation. These were thought to be part of an integrated trophotropic response (the body's opposite response is fight or flight, or ergotropic). Benson and associates therefore surmised that any type of meditation that elicited a trophotropic reaction could be employed rather than TM. He further reasoned that these physiologic alterations appear to be regulated by the hypothalamus as are the ergotropic responses. Therefore the undesirable physiologic effects of stress can be reduced by the relaxation response. Consequently, the relaxation response was studied as a potential therapeutic tool for hypertension. These findings support the theory that environmental and behavioral factors interact to contribute to the development and maintenance of hypertension. This needs further clarification.

Benson and co-workers found the relaxation response to be an effective tool for decreasing blood pressure, particularly with borderline or mildly hypertensive individuals. This lends further credence to the theory that environment and behavior do contribute to the development and progression of hypertension. In recognizing the implications of this new tool on present therapeutic regimens for hypertension, Benson clarifies its usage. He suggests that in a moderate or severe hypertensive, the relaxation response as the single mode of treatment is not sufficient. Drug therapy is effective in controlling the high blood pressure and slowing atherosclerotic disease and, in combination with the relaxation response, reduces the activity of the sympathetic nervous system. The impact of the relaxation response on the cost and side effects of hypertension therapy may prove to be considerable. We agree with these implications and have begun utilizing the relaxation response as an adjunctive mode of therapy for hypertension.

New perspectives regarding the patient's personality as a risk factor have developed. Friedman and Rosenman's personality studies[2] of individuals with cardiovascular disease define a major category of behavior patterns, labeled "type A." This group of personality traits is defined as hostility and a sense of time urgency. These individuals appear to be engaged in a chronic struggle with themselves, people and things (hostility), and time (hurrying, sense of time urgency).

The precise mechanism in type A individuals whereby this stress can effect cardiovascular processes and disease is not known. It has been postulated that changes occur at two levels. The first level is the development of atherosclerosis, which seems to be accelerated due to the increased cholesterol, blood pressure, pulse rate, catecholemines, and tobacco toxicity; over a period of time this damages the vascular walls. The second phase appears to be episodic stresses, which many times can preceed a myocardial infarction. Further studies examining behavioral and psychogenic processes and their etiologic and accelerating effects are needed.

Friedman delineates two methods for recognizing the type A personality profile. The psychomotor manifestations that can be objectively perceived are as follows:

Hostility

Emphatic hand gestures, fist clenching, forceful digital or palm movements
Grating speech pattern—staccato, explosive, unpleasant
Ticlike baring of teeth
Characteristic set of certain facial muscles, particularly around the eyes
Emotional vulnerability

Time urgency

Tense facial muscles
Various muscular movements such as tense posture, frequent blinking of eyes, hastening of general physical movements, knee jiggling, and expiratory sigh
Accelerated speech patterns

The second method involves acquiring data from the history such as being easily irritated in trivial circumstances, extremely opinionated with fixed prejudices, or very self-centered, all of which reflect hostility. Data indicating "hurry sickness" may include a preoccupation about being punctual, infuriation over waiting in line, and performing two activities simultaneously (reading at dinner).

Friedman asserts that recognizing these personality characteristics assists with the identification of high-risk individuals for coronary disease. However, the hypertensive person often effectively conceals these manifestations such that identifying these patterns in the emotional framework is difficult. Friedman utilizes this behavior profile to promote effective therapy by individualizing and personalizing his approach to patients, instructing them in the use of daily medication calendars, and continuously being alert to idiosyncratic or toxic drug reactions which may intensify patients' hostility against the clinician.

Most cardiovascular medical authorities believe that classical therapy to control hypertension cannot be replaced by therapy directed solely at the emotional status of the hypertensive. A patient's personality and emotional patterns may be treated with the fact in mind that this will not decrease blood pressure significantly. If the involved professionals do attempt to change undesirable behavior patterns, this is primarily to prevent coronary disease.

The implications of these theories and findings for nursing are intriguing. Efforts to acquire a comprehensive understanding of each unique patient personality is part of the foundation for assessing, monitoring, and facilitating treatment adherence. As the therapeutic relationship develops with subsequent patient encounters, the assessment of personality and the emotional structure increases in depth and scope. Continuous documentation over a period of time will begin to reflect several salient personality characteristics and behavior patterns. More extensive treatment of the emotional and environmental status of the patient and family are then possible if mutually acceptable. Utilizing the services of a public health nurse, psychologist, social worker, or other health professionals may be indicated.

For counseling purposes a general definition of stress may be as follows:

> Stress is said to occur in any situation that creates an uncomfortable feeling, tension, or strain in the person. Stressful situations usually mean change or adjustment. Each person sees and handles stress differently. Stressful situations may be positive or negative, such as marriage, job change, birth of a child, or death. In these situations or even when hungry or rushing to work, the blood pressure rises and the heart beats faster temporarily. But with hypertension, your blood pressure will rise higher. Your brain, heart, and kidneys need to be protected against that.

People try to relieve the uncomfortable feeling or tension in the following different ways:

- Ignore the situation and not experience the tension
- Switch attention to another activity to relieve the tension
- Face and accept the situation so that it is no longer stressful
- Do nothing but experience the tension
- Seek assistance from other people

However, stress can be handled differently:
1. Look at the problem or stressful situation. Recognize your limits and that you are human.
2. Ask yourself, "What are your responses to the stress? Are they in your best personal and health interests?"
3. Adapt to the stressful problem by thinking about and acting on alternatives or solutions.
4. Learn to relax.

Nutritional considerations[7]

It is noteworthy that twenty-five years ago the complications of hypertension were different from those of today. Congestive heart failure, renal failure, and hemorrhagic strokes were the major problems then, with myocardial infarction or diffuse atherosclerosis occurring less frequently. Currently myocardial infarction is the most common cause of death in the hypertensive population. Thrombotic strokes among white hypertensives and hypertensive renal disease among blacks also are more frequent complications.

Consequently, atherosclerosis as a major contributor to coronary heart disease requires more emphasis. Atherosclerosis accounts for over 1 million deaths a year in the United States. As previously mentioned, hypertension has been found to accelerate the atherosclerotic process. In turn, atherosclerosis accelerates the hypertensive cardiovascular damage and complications.

Excess saturated fats, cholesterol, sodium, alcohol, and caloric consumption have been defined as nutritional risks with hypertension. Obesity, generally defined as excess weight 25% above normal, is an independent risk factor of hypertension. Clearly from available evidence there is a definite relationship between obesity and high blood pressure. The Framingham study demonstrated that obese hypertensives experience twice as much heart disease and premature death than nonobese hypertensives. Individuals who are obese, especially if the weight is gained after maturity, are at substantial risk for cardiovascular disease. This aggravating factor can be monitored and overcome, according to leading weight control authorities and organizations.

There is considerable controversy about the salt content in the American diet, which can be as high as 20 to 30 gm/24 hr. Recent research data have indicated that until the salt intake drops to 5 gm. levels, there is no significant effect on the blood pressure of the hypertensive. Other studies found that the genetic factor of salt sensitivity is significant. Salt-sensitive individuals in both normotensive and hypertensive groups manifested considerable blood pressure and vascular changes in response to salt loading with saline solutions as compared to normal individuals.

We advise slight to moderate salt restriction for our patient populations. This is a preventive measure, since the salt-sensitive individuals are not known, and to avoid the potassium wasting that occurs with a high-salt intake with diuretic therapy.

Recent studies have not established that caffeine in coffee products increases the risk of cardiovascular disease. Furthermore, there is no evidence that de-caffeinated coffee products are safer than regular coffee or tea for patients with hypertension or other forms of cardiovascular diseases.

With this understanding, all hypertensive patients may be provided with diet counseling in terms of the following:

- Salt intake modification
- Intake of potassium-rich foods with diuretic therapy
- Cholesterol intake and saturated fat modification
- Weight control and/or loss

A nutritional history or 24-hour diet recall can be included in the health history interview. Ideally the dietitian or nutritionist on the health care team manages the nutritional therapy according to the physician's objectives. However, in certain health care settings, the nurse is in the best position to manage nutritional therapy as part of the total therapeutic regimen. In this situation the nurse can proceed by obtaining the patient's diet history as follows:

1. Examine daily patterns of food intake in terms of time, amounts, and life-style.
2. Evaluate nutritional intake and balance in terms of the basic four food groups.
3. Explore ethnic, social, and family preferences.
4. Estimate the quantity of sodium and saturated fat intake.
5. Determine food preparation techniques.
6. Acquire an understanding of financial needs and food budgeting practices.
7. Develop an understanding of the psychologic needs and significance of various foods.

With this assessment, a highly individualized approach to diet counseling can be initiated. By expressing positive enthusiasm and interest, with the emphasis on *do's* rather than *don'ts*, patient motivation and subsequent adherence may be greatly enhanced.

The basic four food groups of milk, meat, vegetables and fruit, and breads and cereals can be considered first. The kind, number, and size of servings with alternates and examples of each can be described in detail. Posters, charts, slides, and pamphlets are helpful. Personalizing and individualizing these explanations based on the assessment data is essential.

Following is a suggested patient explanation:

Diet changes are part of your total treatment plan to control your high blood pressure. Basically we would like you to cut down on your salt and salty foods, fatty or high cholesterol foods and keep your weight under control. We may ask you to lose weight, or, if you are on diuretic medicine, to increase your potassium-rich foods. This is the basic diet everyone should follow:

1. Two or more servings of milk or dairy products everyday
2. Two or more servings of meat or substitutes everyday
3. Four or more servings of fruit or vegetables everyday
4. Four or more servings of bread and cereals everyday

Salt-intake modification. Modification of salt intake according to the physician's diet prescriptions can be pursued. The nurse can begin by briefly defining salt, its qualities, and effects as follows:

Salt is a natural chemical, called "sodium chloride," which is found in the human body, foods, and the oceans. Salt is best known as a spice. However, the sodium part of salt acts differently in the human body. There it holds water inside the body. The kidneys are the filters of the body and pass a certain amount of sodium and water out of the body in the urine every day. But the kidneys act slowly. When more salt is eaten than the body needs, more water is held inside the body. This is because the kidneys in hypertensives pass the salt and water out into the urine slowly. This causes the blood pressure to rise further.

The diuretic or water pill the physician has prescribed to control your high blood pressure works with the kidneys to pass more salt and water out of the body in the urine. This is one way to keep the high blood pressure controlled. The diuretic can work best with the kidneys if less salt is eaten on and in your foods. The easiest way to cut down on your salt is not to use salt during your cooking or at the table and eating less salty type foods. This diet plan based on your input and life-style is very helpful.

Following is a brief list of appropriate foods and foods to be avoided. Additional items and food preferences can be incorporated as necessary.

The following high salt foods should be avoided or indulged in only occasionally:

Meat group: Sausage, weiners, ham, bacon, corned beef, luncheon meats or cold cuts, saltpork, smoked fish, herring, sardines, canned meats, "TV" dinners
Dairy group: Cheeses (including processed cheese), buttermilk
Fruit and vegetable group: Olives, pickles, sauerkraut, canned vegetables
Bread and cereal group: Salted crackers, pretzels, rye rolls
Snack foods: Potato chips, pork rinds, salted nuts, salted popcorn
Seasonings: Salt, garlic or onion salt, boullion, soy sauce, Accent, canned soups

The following low-salt foods are encouraged:

Meat and fish group: Poultry, fresh or frozen fish, veal, lamb, pork, beef
Dairy group: Skim milk, low-fat cottage cheese, ice milk
Fresh fruit and vegetable group: Any fresh or frozen foods in the group
Breads and cereals: Most commercial or baked breads or cereals

Snack foods: Sherbet, fruit ice, gelatin, fruit drinks
Seasonings: Garlic, onion, bay leaf, pepper, dill, nutmeg, rosemary, green pepper, lemon juice, others

> Some tips on preparing foods for a low-salt diet are using more fresh or frozen foods and avoiding canned foods, which are high in salt. Also, any leftover cooking liquids can be used with soups or stews.

Patients are told to read the labels of foods when shopping, looking for the salt or sodium content. If the word "sodium" or "salt" is in the first four to five ingredients, they should avoid that food.

Some tips for restaurant eating with a low-salt diet are to eat foods boiled, baked, broiled, or roasted without salted gravies or juices. One can avoid soups and salted or cheesy dressings and carry his own salt substitute or special seasoning.

Emphasis can be placed on enjoying the "real" taste of foods, not just the condiments. Monitoring salt intake of patients at each clinic visit can be accomplished, using the following guidelines:

1. The patient avoids extremely salty foods and adds no salt during cooking or at the table.
2. The patient adds salt in moderation, that is, small amounts during cooking but none at the table.
3. The patient salts food heavily during cooking and at the table.

These are general guidelines for a slight to moderately restricted salt-intake diet.

Increased intake of potassium. In addition to decreasing salt intake for hypertensive patients, the following advice may be provided on increasing potassium intake if they are on diuretic therapy:

> Potassium is a vital mineral in the body, which is chemically a partner to salt. Prescribed diuretics cause more salt and water to pass out of the body to control high blood pressure, but potassium is washed out with the salt. Thus more high-potassium foods must be taken in the diet to replace the loss of potassium. Most fresh fruits and vegetables are high in potassium and should be eaten three to four times a day. Foods such as bananas, oranges, and raisins are especially helpful. Fruit juices are important sources.

A good suggestion is to have one or two fruits every morning along with the diuretic pills. This can be monitored at each visit by asking how many fruit and vegetable servings are eaten a day. Assessing for signs of hypokalemia and comparing serum potassium levels are necessary.

Cholesterol-intake modification. The differentiation between high and low saturated fats is the starting point. Patients can be given the following explanation:

> Generally, all animal fats are saturated, and this includes milk, cream, cheese, butter, beef, and chicken fat. Solid vegetable fats such as shortenings and coconut oils are also saturated. These saturated fats raise blood cholesterol and

fat levels, causing hardening of the arteries. This means that the arteries become stiffer and less movable. Plaques or clumps of fat stick to the walls of blood vessels, making the inside rougher and smaller. This is called "atherosclerosis." Atherosclerosis makes it more difficult for the blood with food and oxygen to pass through and raises the blood pressure. So this is a risk with your high blood pressure. Foods with high saturated fats and cholesterol should then be avoided. Your body produces its own cholesterol, so lots of extra cholesterol in the diet is not needed.

Low saturated or polyunsaturated fats generally include vegetable fats. These polyunsaturated fats lower blood cholesterol and fat levels and are strongly encouraged. Your body does not make polyunsaturated fats and needs them from the diet. Following are some general guidelines for a low saturated fat diet:

1. Use margarine and vegetable oils instead of butter.
2. Avoid gravies, creams, and cheese sauces.
3. Have eggs only three to four times a week. (The number of eggs per week varies with physician's orders.)
4. Drink skim milk and skim milk products.
5. Trim fats from baked, broiled, or boiled meats or poultry.
6. Enjoy poultry, fish, and veal more often. Beef, ham, and pork need to be limited.
7. Avoid fried foods.

When buying foods it is important to read the labels for fat content and to buy foods that are made from polyunsaturated or vegetable fats. Also, buy leaner cuts of meat. Following are tips for low-fat cooking:

1. Trim off as much fat as possible.
2. Broil, roast, or bake your meat using a wire rack so that the fat can drip off.
3. Boil or simmer but immediately remove the meat from the cooking liquid.
4. Do not fry or deep fat fry. You may sauté in a shallow Teflon-coated pan. For soups and gravies, chilling causes the fat to harden, which can then be skimmed off.
5. Cut off all poultry skin.

Monitoring of a low–saturated fat diet is necessary at each clinic visit with periodic laboratory determinations of serum cholesterol and triglycerides. (Refer to the section on patient counseling evaluation in the appendix.)

Weight loss or control. As discussed earlier, patients require counseling about the basic four food groups, salt- and potassium-intake modifications, and low saturated fat diet modifications. If weight loss is indicated, the nurse must jointly explore and determine the need for weight loss sensitively with the patient. Initially resistance may be encountered. Frequently, overweight individuals develop many defenses, rationalizations, and different psychologic processes for ego and body image protection. An honest, empathetic, and supporting relationship is necessary. By explaining that excess weight is a risk factor for hypertension, the focus shifts toward promoting increased patient responsibility for the care of his own body. Various motivational techniques can be employed to help the patient develop insight and to encourage action toward a weight loss goal. Following are some motivational approaches:

1. Action may be directed by utilizing incentives. This may be the incentive

to lower blood pressure, obtain a better job by passing a preemployment physical, or trying to prevent complications from hypertension. Self-directing internal motivations are more desirable and successful. Continuous reinforcement through praise and concrete rewards is necessary to maintain the incentive.

2. Fostering self-confidence in turn nurtures an "I care about myself" feeling. The more a person cares about himself the more apt he will be to undertake constructive action on his behalf.
3. Learning, because it requires changes in either behavior or values, causes anxiety. Depending on the level of anxiety and the individual's coping abilities, a mild level of anxiety can be a motivating factor. The change in value may be related to personal vulnerability from the added risk of obesity for hypertensive complications.
4. Success is an excellent motivator as opposed to failure, which causes a decrease in self-confidence. Small increments of weight loss divided into many short-range goals encourages many smaller successes and negates an overwhelming feeling from a total weight loss goal. Frequent positive reinforcement and appropriate rewards further assist the patient.

With the 24-hour nutritional assessment as a baseline, the nurse can proceed to provide weight loss counseling. Emphasis is placed on the following:

1. The risks of obesity may be explained. Being overweight is an added risk with high blood pressure. More complications such as heart failure, strokes, or kidney disease occur in persons with hypertension who are overweight.
2. The following points about meal planning and scheduling may be emphasized:
   a. Three balanced meals daily
   b. No snacking except for acceptable low calorie foods (individualized lists must be developed)
   c. No meals 4 hours prior to evening sleep
3. Generally, the rate of weight loss should be a pound per week.
4. The preparation and storage of foods are the same as suggested on the low–saturated fat diet. Many questions arise from utilizing two different kinds of food preparation techniques in the same household. Certainly, encouraging proper food preparation for other household members is helpful for preventive purposes. Their participation and support is necessary for the patient to maintain weight control. Therefore it is crucial that diet counseling be provided to both patient and family.
5. Appropriate advice for the management of restaurant eating may be to utilize restaurants that broil foods and to select foods from the menu which most closely follow the low-fat, salt reduction diet.
6. Focus is on *control* and establishing *new eating habits*. Weight will be lost with these new habits. Utilizing the scale as the "iron judge" is not

helpful. If willpower fails and the patient grossly indulges in "forbidden" foods, the nurse can remind the patient that to err is human and to not dwell on it and make excuses, but just proceed positively ahead.

Structured and supportive weight reduction groups can be suggested if the patient and family seem interested. The monitoring at each clinic visit includes the physical parameters of weight; blood pressure; laboratory determinations of blood glucose, cholesterol, and triglycerides as indicated; and changing food intake patterns and control. Further detail is provided in the appendix.

It is important not to cloud or deemphasize the central theme of hypertension treatment but to emphasize to the patient the necessity of following drug therapy and continuing with medical care. By overemphasizing the need to reduce risk factors without determining patient priorities and jointly negotiating therapeutic goals, patients may easily attach considerable significance to these therapeutic adjuncts. More often than not, there is failure to reduce these risks, most of which require considerable life-style changes, and this can precipitate noncompliance with drug therapy and continued medical care.

Complications and treatment regimens

Hypertensive persons must have a basic understanding of the complications of hypertension to make an educated choice regarding their own best interests and the therapeutic regimen. However, this kind of discussion confronts the patient's personal vulnerability and induces anxiety. As discussed in Chapter 7, a mild amount of anxiety can be a motivator, but a severe level of anxiety may be immobilizing. Advice can be more effective if attention is directed at reducing risk factors and emphasizing positive and constructive patient actions.

Following is a simple explanation to describe heart failure as a complication of hypertension:

> High blood pressure can cause heart failure by straining your heart. With high blood pressure your heart must pump against such high pressures that it becomes overworked. The heart muscles become thicker and larger to pump harder and faster. Eventually the heart becomes so thick and weak that it cannot pump enough blood. Worse yet, the blood vessels surrounding the heart may have atherosclerosis (clumps of fat that stick to the blood vessel wall), which further damages the heart and causes a heart failure. Signs of heart failure may be swollen ankles, weight gain, and shortness of breath.

Stroke can be explained to patients as follows:

> High blood pressure can also damage your brain. The pressure of blood causes the blood vessels in the brain to lose their ability to stretch, and they get weak. The blood vessels in the brain are fragile and sensitive. When the blood vessels become too weak, they burst and bleed into the brain. This is a "stroke" and can cause paralysis, which means no feeling or movement of arms and legs. The signs of a stroke may be headache, dizziness, and numbness or weakness in your arms or legs.

Following is a patient explanation for kidney disease:

> The kidneys filter out waste from the blood. High blood pressure damages the tiny blood vessels, and the kidneys can no longer filter out the waste in your blood. Many times there are no signs of kidney disease. This is an extremely serious complication.

Retinal changes can be explained as follows:

> High blood pressure weakens and can damage the blood vessels behind your eye. This is why the physician checks your eyes routinely. Some signs of eye changes may be blurring vision or spots before your eyes. The important point to remember is that hypertension is serious and you need health care. Taking your medicine as ordered and following your physician or nurse's advice will control your high blood pressure.

We do not advocate dwelling on the morbid complications of high blood pressure. However, many patients have questions regarding complications. Clarification may be needed to correct misperceptions the patient or family may have. Again, the emphasis when providing these aspects of high blood pressure counseling is on the positive steps the patient can take to reduce these risks.

Blood pressure fluctuations and trends. Many patients have blood pressure checks between visits at home, health fairs, shopping centers, industries, and schools. It is important to explain fluctuations and trends in blood pressure measurement because patients may discontinue medical management or medication or begin to mistrust the involved professionals if discrepancies in the blood pressure readings occur.

The health care professional needs to emphasize that blood pressure varies from moment to moment and from activity to activity, and there is a diurnal pattern that is lower in the morning and rises until early evening. Anxiety, apprehension, pain, and sudden loud noises may affect the blood pressure on a short-term basis. The patient must be informed of his blood pressure goal with therapy and the usual range of fluctuation to be expected.

Methods of treatment. At the initial visit an orientation to clinic procedures and patient care services may be provided to the patient and family. This minimizes anxiety and clarifies patient expectations.

The steps in the process of the patient's individualized care need clarification and reinforcement frequently. Patient participation and responsibility for the therapeutic "contract" is essential. Each aspect of therapy for hypertension control is fully described to the patient and family.

The patient must know the following about antihypertensive drug therapy:

1. The patient can be told the goals of therapy, that is, what his controlled blood pressure is expected to be and what his current blood pressure is at each clinic visit in relation to that goal.
2. The medications control but do not cure high blood pressure. Therapy is lifelong.

3. The name, type of drug, how it works, and the rationale for its use.
4. The time of day and pills to take. Written reinforcement is helpful.
5. Changes or side effects may occur for a short time or sometimes longer as his body and blood pressure are adjusting to the medication. Request that the patient tell his physician or nurse about any problems or changes being experienced.
6. Each person's body acts in a unique way with each medicine, and the drugs may be changed or switched until his blood pressure is controlled adequately.
7. It is necessary to take the drugs every day as ordered.
8. The patient should never stop taking the medications without the physician or nurse's advice.
9. All medications taken since the last appointment can be brought to the clinic at each visit. This is because the physician or nurse wants to make sure that the patient is taking the right medication in the right way. In addition, occasionally between clinic visits a patient may become ill and take other medications that the physician or nurse need to know about.
10. The patient should avoid taking other medications without telling the physician or nurse because these may interfere with the action of the blood pressure medication.
11. With high blood pressure, the physician may prescribe several kinds of medicines to be taken every day. This "team" of medicines works well to control the patient's hypertension. Besides diuretics, the other members of this team of medicines that may be prescribed are nerve blockers and vasodilators.

More specific counseling regarding pertinent aspects of drug therapy is described in Chapter 5 and Appendix B.

SUMMARY

The nurse's role in hypertension control has expanded dramatically. The patient education component is strategic in facilitating entry into the health care system and increasing adherence to treatment. The counseling process for hypertension control has two major phases. The blood pressure screening procedure may be utilized not only as a hypertension detection system but also as an educational tool. The second phase of the counseling process deals with the treatment of the hypertensive individual and his family. Counseling focuses on treatment aspects and the adaptation by the patient to a long-term illness. Primarily, predisposing factors, nutritional considerations, complications, and treatment aspects are emphasized.

The simple explanations presented for patient understanding can readily be adapted, expanded, or sophisticated to meet patient and family needs and educational abilities. Counseling for multiple predisposing and risk factors is a long process, requiring continuous reinforcement. Frequently, patients and families become confused regarding priorities of hypertension therapy and what is expected of them if the nurse does not repeatedly clarify these aspects in simple terms.

SUGGESTED READINGS

1. Benson, H.: The relaxation response, New York, 1975, The William Morrow Co.
2. Friedman, M.: The psychological profile of a hypertensive patient: an explanation of his therapeutic response, Am. Heart Assoc. Bull., No. 5008A, 1975.
3. Kannel, W. B., et al.: Epidemiologic assessment of the role of blood pressure in stroke: the Framingham study, J.A.M.A. **214:**301-310, 1970.
4. Kannel, W. B., et al.: Role of blood pressure in the development of congestive heart failure: the Framingham study, N. Engl. J. Med. **287:**781-787, 1972.
5. Kaplan, N.: Your blood pressure: the most deadly high, New York, 1974, Medcom Press, Inc.
6. Klatsky, A. L., et al.: Alcohol consumption and blood pressure: Kaiser-Permanente multiphasic health examination data, N. Engl. J. Med. **296:**1194-1199, 1977.
7. Margie, J. O., and Hunt, J. C.: Living with high blood pressure: the hypertension diet cookbook, Bloomfield, N. J., 1978, HLS Press, Inc.
8. Miller, N. E.: Applications of learning and biofeedback to psychiatry and medicine. In Freedman, A. M., Kaplan, H. I., and Sadock, B. J., editors: Comprehensive textbook of psychiatry, Baltimore, 1975, The Williams & Wilkins Co.
9. Pohl, M. L.: Teaching function of the nurse practitioner, Dubuque, Iowa, 1968, William C. Brown Co., Publishers.
10. Redman, B. K.: The process of patient teaching in nursing, St. Louis, 1972, The C. V. Mosby Co.
11. Skinner, B. F.: Behavior of organisms, New York, 1938, Appleton-Century-Crofts.
12. The Hypertension Handbook, West Point, Pa., 1974, published by Merck, Sharp & Dohme in cooperation with the National High Blood Pressure Education Program.

CHAPTER 7

Compliance with antihypertensive therapy

DEFINITIONS[17]

Patient "compliance," or "adherence," can be generally defined as maintenance of an assigned therapeutic regimen. "Noncompliance" is said to exist when the patient does not adhere to the prescribed therapeutic regimen.

Considerable variation exists in the functional definitions of compliance and the determination of the point at which compliance stops and noncompliance begins. There are three general approaches to the measurement of compliance:

1. *Biologic basis*, a direct approach that includes ascertaining blood or urinary excretion levels of medications, metabolites, or markers
2. *Arbitrary cutoff points*, which are usually decided on a statistical basis or are suggested by earlier studies but that have no biologic or behavioral validity
3. *Indirect measures* such as pill counts (comparing amount of medication prescribed to amount remaining in patient's bottle) and prescription refills, patient interview (eliciting the patient's estimate of his own compliance), therapeutic or preventive results of the regimen, incidental metabolic effects (measurement of serum potassium levels in hypertensives who take prescribed thiazides), and the clinician's estimates

Noncompliance may occur through a variety of mechanisms and is manifested by behavior patterns such as delay in acquiring medical care, avoiding preventive community programs (blood pressure screening), appointment and medication failures, and resisting and/or not maintaining the prescribed therapeutic regimen. The therapeutic regimen may include directions that are additive to the patient's life-style, such as medications or exercise, and restrictive, such as diet and activity levels. With each type of noncompliance, clinical setting, and individuals involved, the measurement parameters of noncompliance are different. What is important is whether the purpose of the noncompliance measurements is for research or clinical services. If for research, measurement parameters are stringent and precise; if for clinical service, less detail is necessary. Generally, any appropriate measurement parameters for noncompliance in a clinical setting that reasonably predict and identify an acceptable number of noncompliers in the treated population are sufficient.

We have designed an operational definition of noncompliance for our clinical settings. These definitions are derived from several theoretical models for noncompliance, since no singular theoretical framework fully explains or details strategies for noncompliance. Further study and qualification is necessary and in process.

Noncompliance is indirectly measured as follows:

I. Primary parameters
   A. Sustained or progressively elevated blood pressure levels in the absence of secondary causes, complications, volume expansion, and high stress levels
   B. Failure to take medications as prescribed
   C. Missing scheduled appointments or dropping out of treatment
   D. Failure to interact with the clinician or interacting without mutual satisfactory results
      1. Mutual expectations not satisfied and/or questions not answered
      2. Lack of mutual agreement about therapeutic plans and goals
      3. Failure to report medication side effects and other related problems of therapy and adherence

II. Secondary parameters
   A. Lack of modification of identified risk factors as jointly agreed on
      1. Maintenance of excess weight or weight gain and the maintenance of high-salt, cholesterol, and caloric intake
      2. Unchanged or increased smoking habits
      3. Unchanged or increased alcohol intake
      4. Lack of daily exercise and relaxation routine
   B. Failure to demonstrate readiness or acceptance to adhere to a therapeutic regimen
      1. General attitude and response to health professionals and care is hostile, antagonistic, or withdrawn
      2. Refusal to ask questions and/or participate in educational and other clinic services
      3. Family participation and support is lacking in cases when appropriate
      4. Does not appear to have a consistent motivational level

A detailed discussion of these parameters of noncompliance is presented later in the section on monitoring compliance.

MAGNITUDE OF NONCOMPLIANCE

The medical and nursing professions within the past decade have begun to formally recognize the pervasive problem of noncompliance with therapeutic regimens. The paradox is that the clinician is frequently the last to know when the patient is noncompliant. Although the health care provider may sense noncompliance in particular patients, it is almost always underestimated.

Historically the commonly used antihypertensive medications were not available until the 1950s to 1960s. About that time the magnitude of the problem of hypertension was realized. The Veteran's Administration Cooperative Study published in 1967 and 1970 distinctly defined the scientific basis for the treatment of moderate and severe hypertension. During the 1970s, noncompliance with hypertension therapy was first recognized as a considerable problem preventing successful treatment. The results of surveys by Wilber,[21] Stamler,[19] and Shoenberger and others[18] correlate with the Milwaukee Blood Pressure Program data (Figs. 1 to 3), which reveal large numbers of hypertensives who are either untreated or uncontrolled.

The Milwaukee Blood Pressure Program has a physician follow-up system that has been in existence about three years since the program's inception. This consists of periodically contacting physicians for follow-up data on referred suspected hypertensives detected through our blood pressure screening process. The cumulative results are as follows:

Compliance (as judged by continued therapy) (N = 1160)		Compliance (as judged by blood pressure control) (N = 1310)	
Continued drug therapy	89%	Patients lost to follow-up	7%
Drug stopped by patient	8.8%	Uncontrolled blood pressure	26%
Drug stopped by physician	2.2%	Controlled blood pressure	67%

This demonstrates the extent of compliance and noncompliance with therapy in a metropolitan community and the degree of blood pressure control that physicians are achieving. Remarkably, physicians estimated that 89% are continuing the drug treatment, but only 67% had controlled blood pressure.

Most studies indicate that one-third of patients fail to comply with physician's orders. Twenty percent of patients with symptomatic disease do not keep their appointments, and more than 50% do not follow medication orders. Asymptomatic patients have 50% appointment failures and even greater medication failures. Long-term prophylactic therapy as in rheumatic fever has compliance rates of approximately 40% or less. In terms of noncompliance with hypertension treatment, the findings of most studies parallel the general literature review. Approximately a third of patients take their medicines conscientiously, one third occasionally, and one third only rarely.

Table 3. Results of counseling and treatment at Milwaukee County Downtown Medical and Health Services Hypertension Clinic (N = 1000 patients)

	Initial evaluation (%)	Nine-month follow-up evaluation (%)
Smoking		
None or occasional	45	51
<1 pack/day	25	30
≥1 pack/day	30	19
Alcohol consumption		
None or occasional	50	63
Weekends only	27	23
Daily	12	11
Heavy	11	3
Body weight		
Normal	19	18
<20% overweight	39	40
≥20% overweight	42	42
Blood pressure level		
Normal	9	43
Mild hypertension	41	42
Moderate hypertension	28	11
Severe hypertension	22	4

Results of counseling and treatment services in our hypertension clinic are shown in Table 3. Several salient trends can be noted. Counseling regarding smoking and alcohol consumption had a desirable effect in that patients moved from severe to milder categories. However, body weight results did not change. This correlates with other findings in the literature, which indicate that dietary and life-style modifications are exceedingly difficult to effect and maintain. Substantial blood pressure control was achieved.

REASONS FOR NONCOMPLIANCE

There is no one proven theoretical model for noncompliance. Following is a summary of current theories on noncompliance. One can draw implications where relevant and desirable. At the end of the chapter a list of suggested readings is provided from which most of the theories and data are extracted.

Sociologic and demographic considerations

Numerous sociologic and demographic studies directed at the causes of noncompliance have failed to delineate these. Both compliance and noncompliance appear to be prevalent in all social and demographic levels.

Sociodemographic studies attempt to describe the nature and characteristics of segments of the hypertensive population and suggest some generalizations with respect to the findings. The problem is that each variable such as income, sex, age, race, or religion is encompassing and closely interwoven with other variables. For example, marital status reflects differences in age, income, stress, and others. It is not feasible to differentiate which will be the stronger predictor for compliance. Demographic factors correlate more with how individuals utilize health care facilities rather than compliance with prescribed therapy. The indigent black population utilizes health care facilities differently than affluent whites. We believe that the work site setting studies on hypertension control will address this issue. In summary, the sociodemographic approach as a singular method of study has not been sufficient to define the predictors of noncompliance.

Psychologic factors

In Chapter 6, Friedman's attempts to objectively note various behavior patterns and personality traits predicting high risk personalities for cardiovascular disease were presented. However, studies to investigate the correlation between adherence to cardiovascular disease therapy and these type A individuals are necessary. A similar approach to describe personality traits as predictors for compliance has employed the Minnesota Multiphasic Personality Inventory. This attempts to measure traits such as dependency, authoritarianism, self-esteem, impulsivity, and others but has not rendered consistent associations with compliance.

The relationship of stress and anxiety to hypertension and the need for clarification of its causes, aggravating effects, and possible influences on compliance was previously discussed in Chapter 6. It does seem reasonable that hypertension therapy should include provisions for stress reduction.

In Sackett and Haynes' exhaustive review of the compliance literature,[17] psychologic factors such as active-versus-passive orientation, self-esteem levels, acting-out behavior, crisis, alienation, loneliness, intelligence, educational levels, and others were studied, but the findings were inconclusive.

Patient factors in noncompliance

Perceptions, motivations, and priorities. Several interesting studies reveal that noncompliant individuals perceive themselves as less vulnerable to potential or present illness. Comparing noncompliers with compliers, the diagnosis being the same, the noncompliers perception of the severity and seriousness of the disease problem was less than the physician's evaluation of it. We think this perception is extremely important for compliance.

Studies conducted on cardiac patients with disturbed perceptions of their present therapeutic and rehabilitative regimen indicated that these individuals utilized direct activity to decrease frustration or externalization. Their immaturity, lack of receptivity, firm assertions of independence, defensiveness, and arrogant outspokenness were identified. Although these observations are subjective in nature, their significance as possible manifestations of distorted perceptions may have implications for noncompliance.

In addition, noncompliers have been found to be less concerned with their health and less confident in modern medical management. One study pinpointed that a patients' conscious intention to adhere to the prescribed regimen immediately after a clinic visit is an indication for future compliance. Of patients in this study, 40% stated that their intention was never to comply. In terms of the patient's confidence in the accuracy of the diagnosis, one study evaluated the degree to which patients agreed with the physician's decision and their appraisal of the certainty of his decisions. The results successfully predicted subsequent compliance. We have also found this to be true. When patients transfer from their physician to the nurse clinic, after initial evaluation and treatment, their degree of confidence in the physician's diagnosis and his certainty is positively associated with compliance. Besides treatment dropout, patients who for one reason or another have little confidence in the diagnosis or the certainty of the physician decisions most frequently refuse medication therapy. However, many of these individuals have periodic blood pressure checks or consider risk factor modification.

The perceived severity of the disease process is a determining factor for compliance. Based on Becker and others' health belief model,[1,2] even though the individual perceives vulnerability, he will not take action without also believing that the disease will cause bodily or social harm. The perceived severity of an illness being presently experienced consistently predicted compliance. In this case, an explanation may be that since a diagnosis is made and the patient is experiencing symptoms, this reality effect on perceived severity motivates the patient to comply. This appears to correlate only during the initial phase of treatment. Once a patient "feels better," there is subsequent noncompliance. We agree with these findings and suggest the significant implications for hypertension therapy that is usually prescribed on a long-term basis to a relatively asymptomatic population. Studies correlating perceived severity and the subsequent preventive measures are inconclusive. Hence, for asymptomatic individuals to have annual blood pressure checks for hypertension, it appears that an appropriate degree of perceived severity is necessary.

Four major patterns of health behavior have been described as follows:

1. *Preventive health behavior* in which the individual feels well or "healthy" and undertakes actions to prevent illness or determine its asymptomatic presence. An example would be the annual blood pressure check.
2. *Illness health behavior* in which the individual "feels sick" and undertakes actions to have the illness evaluated and treated. The undetected hypertensive person with frequent occipital morning onset headaches who seeks medical care is an example.
3. *Sick role behavior* in which actions are undertaken by the treated patient

to "get well" or resume varying levels of functioning. This may be illustrated by the recovering stroke (hypertensive) patient participating in a rehabilitation program.

4. *At-risk behavior* by means of which a healthy individual takes steps to modify or minimize his risk factors or predisposition to a disease. For example, the normotensive overweight smoker with a strong family history of hypertension and cardiac complications who joins weight loss and anti-smoking classes.

The preventive and at-risk health behaviors are somewhat similar. These roles in varying degrees have privileges or social support accompanying their duties and have a highly flexible or nonspecific time framework to accomplish their goals. Illness health behavior and sick role behavior do merit privileges such as bed rest, special attention, and work and social obligation release.

Current research has not yet defined the predictors of at-risk behavior. However, when an individual engages in these types of behaviors, they may be assessed; the nurse can examine in retrospect the interrelated predisposing influences leading the individual to that behavior. These interrelated predisposing influences can be cultivated and maximized to facilitate and maintain healthy behaviors through appropriate education, behavior modification, and social support interventions.

The traditional approach of predicting compliance has been from the health belief model, which is based on motivational theory. The discussion so far has addressed the set of factors concerning the value of reducing the threat of illness by means of an individual's perceptions of one's vulnerability and susceptibility and the severity of the disease process. Another major category of predictors in the health belief model is specific patient *motivation*. This impetus for action has been measured in terms of the patient's conscious intentions to adhere and the influence of symptoms and disease threats. Specific patient motivations such as a genuine concern about health, previous utilization of preventive health services, the degree of compliance with other prescribed therapies, and again the confidence in and attitude toward the medical authority have been positively associated with compliance.

We agree that the degree of control over health matters and the priorities of the individual may be significant as Caplan and co-workers[5] suggest. The crucial consideration is that the therapeutic goals and steps to achieve those goals, such as weight loss or the elimination of smoking, be derived from the individual's motives and priorities. The goals of blood pressure control and weight loss may be related to motives other than self-preservation such as obtaining new employment (self-image–self-esteem motives). Although as health professionals we can affect the steps and impediments to attaining the goal, the motives that establish the goal are not readily alterable.

Motives and their striving activities compete. For example, when a hypertensive patient is prescribed medications, he must decide whether to take them. In actuality he must choose which of his motives is strongest, most relevant, and valued at that time. This is an extremely important consideration. It appears that compliant behaviors must be *useful* as steps toward valued and relevant goals and more *beneficial* (time, effort, cost) than other activities. Health care providers may not necessarily agree with their patients' perceptions about the value, relevance, usefulness, and benefits of compliant behaviors. However, we respect and make every attempt to understand, incorporate, and possibly alter those perceptions as a basis for constructing an individualized therapeutic regimen.

Medications and therapeutic regimens. Behavioral changes on the part of the patient are a consequence of a therapeutic regimen. Compliance will more often be with those areas of the therapeutic regimen that are simple, easiest, and least disruptive to preexisting behavior and life-style. Therefore only certain portions of the regimen may be adopted, depending on the degree of behavioral changes required.

Therapies that require passive participation on the patient's part have better adherence rates. In contrast, there is a marked gradient of difference in noncompliance rates with patients who must actively participate in treatment, especially in terms of changing behavioral habits. This includes diet, smoking, alcohol consumption, and job-related activities. Data presented in Table 3 support these impressions.

The duration and expense of the prescribed therapy for the most part are inversely correlated with compliance. It appears that minimizing the cost and time framework for treatment enhances adherence rates. In our opinion, this has tremendous implications for hypertension treatment in that the drug therapy is long-term. Many patients resist long-term drug therapy. They believe that therapy for a few months' duration will "cure" the hypertension. In addition, some patients object to the cost of the drugs.

There is no clear evidence regarding the size and frequency of dosage each day as affecting compliance. However, our use of combination tablets and minimizing the frequency of daily dosages have enhanced compliance. Addition of drugs to the regimen reduces compliance. One study specifically found increased drug default when potassium and diuretic medication were added to a digoxin regimen. We have also observed adherence problems when employing more than two drugs in the antihypertensive regimen.

The type and form of medications have not been conclusively found to affect compliance.

In terms of side effects, little data are available in the literature examining the possible association with noncompliance. One study of hypertensive patients found side effects were not a significant determinant. In our experience, side effects have been found to affect adherence, although not significantly. This has been more frequent with drugs that produce dizziness, fatigue, impotence, and gastric disturbances, especially if these effects interfere with job or personal activities.

A pivotal point is that noncompliers usually do not volunteer that information to the clinician. Therefore it follows that problems with side effects may not be revealed to the clinician. We have found this to be true after asking specific questions in this regard.

In addition to the aforementioned factors, the safety dispensers for medications have been found to decrease compliance.

As discussed previously, the patient perceptions regarding the therapeutic regimen that affect compliance are as follows:

1. The relative safety of the prescribed regimen
2. The effectiveness and benefits of the regimen in terms of preventing, delaying, or curing illness and the patient's confidence in the physician's diagnosis and modern health care

The clinician's attitude toward and confidence in the prescribed therapy is important. Anticipating what the patient can expect in terms of possible changes with therapy can allay the patient's concern regarding the safety of the regimen. Furthermore, we believe that presenting new changes to the patient as *expected temporary adjustments* to therapy minimizes their threat. The patient is reassured that his body and blood pressure need time to adjust to the therapy and that the clinician is available to discuss problems and alter plans as needed. In addition, side effects and their management are clearly differentiated from expected temporary adjustments.

Complying with one or more of the therapies prescribed in the total regimen appears to positively predict adherence with other facets of the regimen. The relationship between appointment attendance and adherence to the prescribed regimen is unclear. We have noted that appointment failures are usually associated with medication failures. Unfortunately the converse cannot be assumed for patients keeping appointments.

There has been little research in terms of the patient collaborating with the clinician in selecting therapeutic strategies from the possible appropriate alternatives. One study indicated that the patient must believe that it is valid and reasonable to participate, that he has the capability to make decisions, and that the facets of the therapeutic regimen and contract are of personal importance. Many of our patients are pleasantly surprised when asked, for example, which of two possible therapeutic alternatives they would prefer. However, we believe that if the patient is not given the appropriate information, his ability to make decisions is impaired.

Family participation. Noncompliance is more prevalent among those individuals with unstable or indifferent families and those living alone. Social and emotional support is necessary for compliance. This enhances self-confidence and decreases psychologic and physical strains. Studies have revealed an increase in the risk of coronary disease among individuals grieving the loss of a loved one by death, rejection, or indifference or having job-related rejection. However, we have noted that the degree of support needs to be individualized so as not to threaten autonomy. Also, continuity of care by the same clinician facilitates the therapist's delivery and the patient's reception of support.

Health education. The data regarding the relationship between the patient's knowledge of his disease process and treatment and the adherence rates are conflicting.[4,17,20] Perhaps the problem lies in questionable research methodology, behavioral determinants, or use of educational principles.

The assumption that if individuals are informed they will undertake the suggested constructive actions appears to be false. There is a vast gulf between knowing and doing. In our opinion, what seems to be important is the patient and family's perception of, value of, and participation in the educational process. They have the right and responsibility to make decisions about health care and adherence. Therefore they must know the relevant information.

Clearly delineated written and verbal instructions and expectations enhance compliance. Two studies examining patient recall on physician's instructions revealed that over half of the instructions were quickly forgotten and subsequently accompanied by varied levels of anxiety. Recall is best with a precise and brief list of instructions.

Fear arousal messages as a tool for compliance has been studied with conflicting results. Janis' review[14] of the literature on fear content in therapeutic messages found no relationship between high fear levels and the patient's disposition to adhere. Podell[16] summarizes the mechanisms by which fear provokes behavioral changes. Upon fear stimulation, the individual becomes vigilant. The person is circumspect and scrutinizes the environment for the type, degree, and proximity of the threat and resources and avenues to keep the threat distant. Feelings of stress and strain, and a desire for support and comfort are evoked. At this point, the individual is hypersuggestible, and dependent on authorities with solutions minimizing the threat and anxiety. There are numerous behavioral responses. The individual may act on the suggested solution (adaptive), pursue alternatives, or ignore the threat. Podell purports that the third behavioral response (fear avoidance) may be a primary cause of noncompliance.

An important consideration is that low fear levels increase the individual's attention to the problem; however, high levels are incapacitating, decreasing the person's ability to adhere. As explained in Chapter 6, we utilize highly individualized levels of fear messages and have found this approach to be most useful and humanistic. In our experience, the fear-evoking message must always be accompanied with an emphasis on the positive steps and benefits of modification that the patient can undertake.

The few studies examining the effects of the various teaching strategies such as group sessions, individual counseling, programmed instruction, and demonstration yield weak correlations with compliance. Our experience, on the other hand, indicates that continuously employing a variety of individualized teaching approaches improves patient awareness and compliance.

Clinician factors in noncompliance

Perceptions, motivations, and priorities. Caron and Roth[6,7] compared physicians' estimation of antacid use by their patients with the number of medication bottles used. Physicians overestimated compliance by 46%. As previously discussed, the Milwaukee Blood Pressure Program data revealed that private physicians estimated 89% of their patients were continuing with the prescribed treatment.

The other significant study was that of Davis,[8,9] who again documented considerable discrepancy. Over half the physicians estimated that almost all their patient population followed the prescribed regimen, and only 7% indicated that less than one half adhered. The causes for noncompliance as stated by the physicians were patient's personality (66%), patient's inability to comprehend the medical advice (8%), and the physician's attitude (26%). The following physicians' actions in order of their use were documented: detailed explanation of the prescribed regimen, influence through a convincing credible appeal, threats, and case referral or withdrawal. Davis' findings suggest one cause of the physicians' overestimates of adherence: the degree of ego investment by a physician in the relationship with the patient. Believing that the patient is adhering to his regimen and recognizing his authority are positive reinforcements; however, these may decrease the ability to determine patient noncompliance.

Regarding the clinician's motivation and priorities, authorities such as Moser and Finnerty suggest several contributing factors to physician noncompliance.[13] Performing a blood pressure measurement is presently not always a routine part of the physician's examination. This implies that blood pressure is of minor importance, and this can be readily perceived by the patient and consequently instilled as an appropriate value. Moreover, many physicians do not perceive the seriousness of mild blood pressure elevations and therefore do not treat these cases.

Physicians have been trained to respond to symptoms and complaints. Since hypertension is an asymptomatic disease, the patient usually does not complain or ask the physician for help. The physician does not therefore receive reinforcement from prevention or early aggressive treatment in the mild stages. Fortunately, medical school curricula are now being changed to incorporate the preventive emphasis.

As discussed earlier, there is also a difference in priorities between the patient and the physician. The clinician's priorities may be to decrease the blood pressure, whereas the patient may be concerned with the treatment cost and interference with job activities.

Interactional considerations. We strongly agree with the universal consensus that the quality of the clinician-patient interaction is crucial for compliance.[3,11,12,15] However, there are conflicting opinions about the various aspects of influences on and predictors of this relationship. The clinician who conveys interest, friendliness, warmth, and an understanding of the patient's concerns has been found to increase patient satisfaction, but not necessarily adherence. A disagreeable or offensive clinician approach negatively affects patient satisfaction and cooperation. A long-lasting relationship in which there is good rapport and open and honest communication between patient and clinician affects compliance positively.

Francis and co-workers[10] found that patients with high levels of satisfaction are more likely to comply. The mechanism is purported to be that the positive feelings about himself (patient) and his compliant behavior are reflected as feelings of satisfaction with the clinician and the interaction. They also suggest that the physician's appraisal of the illness and its health threat affect patient perception more than patient motivation. The physician's failure to communicate rather than a patient's inability to comprehend generates dissatisfaction and noncompliance at higher rates.

Davis' extensive analysis of physician-patient interaction yielded evidence that noncompliance can be attributed to difficult and disturbed communication.[8,9] This was demonstrated when physicians were formal and disdaining, there were attempts by both the physician and patient to control one another with lack of agreement, and tension was not discharged. Furthermore, noncompliance resulted in situations in which dictatorial patients were treated by lenient physicians and in those in which the physician did not return feedback after obtaining detailed data from the patient.

Podell[16] has elaborated on Svartstad's unpublished study of the physician-patient encounter. Approximately one third of noncompliers had difficulty determining the physician's expectations of what should be done with the prescribed medication. When the physician provided detailed instructions, there was a demonstrable increase in patient comprehension and adherence. The physician imparted more information and explanation when actively questioned. Of Svartstad's population, 60% could not later define terms discussed at the physician encounter such as high blood pressure, hypertension, sodium, and others. This supports the findings of other studies in which patients fail to convey their misunderstanding to the physician.

Svartstad further demonstrated that physicians frequently prevented or dissuaded patient communication or questions by means of a behavioral index of approachability. She observed the following distancing maneuvers on the physician's part: conspicuous surveying of the clock and waiting room; indistinct or inarticulate murmuring; disregarding, stopping, or interrupting patient communication; telephone interruptions; and initiating the interaction by receiving a disease rather than a person ("What's the problem?" as opposed to "How are you?").

Several techniques that physicians employed to promote compliance were successful. These included describing the need and rationale for the medicine (appeal to the patient's reason), focusing on and reinforcing the regimen (the need for refilling prescriptions), and utilizing medical authority ("Take this prescription" versus "Do you want this medicine?"). Compliance was also enhanced with a high monitoring approach by the physician (specifically questioning adherence and patient problems with the regimen). We have been employing these techniques with successful results.

The study of Podell and Kent on compliance with hypertension therapy in a suburban family practice setting yielded informative results.[16] Supporting other studies, medication side effects were not found to be a significant influence. The important findings were that the physicians contributed to noncompliance by failing to aggressively prescribe for hypertension control. Physicians failed to increase dosages in response to patient anxiety and did not prescribe drug therapy because the patient's obesity was the "obvious source" of the blood pressure problem. They failed to aggressively treat when patients indicated definite opposition. Finally, some physicians submitted to patient objections without a specified reason.

The degree to which patients affect and determine physician behavior during the therapeutic interaction appears to be considerable. Podell further elaborated on the patient's psychologic avoidance and rationalizations opposing more aggressive therapy. The physician's response after several such encounters was to assume a more lenient posture. Also, this implied agreement continued and was a significant aspect of a long-term relationship, despite inadequately controlled blood pressure. Based on Davis' work, Podell suggested that a mild or minimally authoritative physician allows the patient to be overtly opposed to his advice. In contrast, the physician who projects a high level of authority elicits more covert patient opposition such as medication and appointment failures.

In terms of the causes for the patient's denial, Podell's findings were consistent with perceived vulnerability, susceptibility, and severity as discussed earlier. Fear of death and the threat to body and self-image also were stated or implied causes. The degree of patient independence in the therapeutic relationship again appeared to be a significant factor. In the therapeutic relationship the patient assumes a more dependent position and submits to the limits of his control. Consequently, the degree of patient independence needs to be individualized, since some individuals may attempt a variety of distancing maneuvers.

MONITORING COMPLIANCE

The monitoring of compliance with the prescribed therapeutic regimen is incorporated as an integral part of each visit to our clinic. Initially the approach is a high monitoring strategy. Later, once comfortably settled into a mutually satisfying therapeutic relationship with consistent blood pressure control and motivational levels, a lower-key, highly individualized monitoring strategy is employed.

We do not utilize direct parameters for measuring compliance such as biologic markers and metabolites. Our measures are indirect and the cutoff point at which compliance stops and noncompliance begins is negotiable, since each patient and family is viewed and treated on an individual basis. We do not quantify (assign points) to each parameter in our operational definition of noncompliance, described earlier, to "add up" to a diagnosis of noncompliance. Indirect measures are used as flexible and negotiable guidelines to evaluate patient noncompliance and determine the appropriate strategies.

With that frame of reference, we will discuss point by point how the parameters of our operational definition of noncompliance are monitored. Since this definition is so encompassing, various aspects are discussed in other chapters.

The evaluation of sustained or progressively elevated blood pressure levels in terms of secondary causes, complications, volume expansion, and high stress levels is presented in Chapters 4 and 5. When the evaluation excludes those causes, noncompliance with the prescribed regimen is strongly suspected.

To further assess, we share with the patient and family his blood pressure "track record" and ask why he thinks his blood pressure is elevated today or has progressively risen. The patient's perceptions, insights, feelings, and identified contributors to the elevated blood pressure are occasionally surprising and correct. Responses such as admitting medication failures due to insomnia or impotence, an increase in alcohol and salt intake, intrapersonal difficulties, and unemployment are common. Other patients state that they do not know why their blood pressure is elevated. We ask "why" questions with discretion, since these ask the patient to identify a cause that he usually does not know. In addition, the patient may be maneuvered into agreeing with the clinician and selecting one contributory factor at the expense of other factors. Furthermore, we have found that inner-city clientele usually do not think in introspective terms, and this line of questioning may be frustrating.

Our attitude toward noncompliant behavior is nonjudgmental or "no fault." Clinician and patient mutually collaborate in the relationship and decision making and share mutual responsibility for its outcomes. Therefore we do not blame or label patients for "bad" or noncompliant behaviors.

In terms of assessing whether the medication is taken as prescribed, we perform a rough estimate of compliance by comparing the number of pills dispensed with pills remaining in the prescription bottles. We do not methodically count pills in the patient's presence but estimate roughly. Positive reinforcement is given for remembering to bring the medication bottles to the clinic. We also consult the pharmacist as necessary. It is helpful to compare the expected degree of blood pressure control with the current blood pressure level; the anticipated metabolic effects of the medication with present serum potassium, uric acid, and blood sugar levels; and the anticipated side effects such as orthostatic hypotension, dizziness, impotence, or others with the patient's present complaints.

We ask specific questions to elicit both positive and negative feedback about the medication regimen, such as the names, frequency, times of day, and numbers of pills taken. We also ask how many times a week the patient forgets to take his medicine and when he forgets most often and why then. If a medication calendar is kept, it is reviewed at the time of each visit. In addition, the patient is asked if he takes the medication in conjunction with a specific daily activity (e.g., brushing his teeth in the morning). We elicit detailed feedback regarding any changes or difficulties. Information is elicited with regard to the expense of the prescriptions in terms of the patient's ability to pay and obtain the full prescribed quantities. Furthermore, the patient and family are asked what the medication is, how it works, and why he is taking it to assess their level of understanding and perceptions about the regimen.

When a scheduled appointment is missed, the outreach system is put into effect as described in Chapter 8. Every attempt is made to ascertain the reason why the patient did not attend the clinic by means of personal telephone calls, home visits, and letters. Community health and occupational health nurse collaboration is extremely effective in terms of reaching, monitoring, and assisting the noncomplier in his home and work setting. We also convey that if there are shortcomings in the clinic organization or personnel that affect the attendance, we would like to know. We care and are willing to change to meet their needs or address their problems, but we need to know those problems and needs. Patients are assured of our confidence and support and that there will be no punitive effects. If a patient drops out of treatment, the outreach system is continued and he is informed that he may return at any time for treatment. We request that the patient inform us if he is being treated elsewhere, so that we are assured he is receiving medical care.

In terms of a patient who is not interacting with the clinician or interacting without satisfactory results, we first assess the individual personality traits and their influence and implications for compliance. Is the patient hostile, aggressive, anxious, neurotic, paranoid, or hypochondriac? Does the patient have traits such as negative attitudes toward authority figures, inappropriate dependency, exaggerated autonomy, risk-taking and acting-out behaviors, or low self-esteem? To what degree are these traits or behaviors present? Possible influences and implications for compliance can be estimated by determining the patient's previous history of compliance with medical regimens. For example, a patient who is aggressive, displays negative attitudes toward authority figures, and did not adhere to a previously prescribed regimen is a strong risk for noncompliance. His negative energy and behavior can be channeled into mutual participation and decision making in the clinician-patient interaction.

Medication calendars may not be of value in the extremely anxious or neurotic patient. Hypochondriac or dependent persons are not viewed as candidates for home blood pressure measurements.

Next we attempt to assess how these traits and behaviors are accepted within and influence the family or social support. What type and degree of accommodations are made by the family for these traits and behaviors? When and what support and limits are employed? This may suggest to the clinician what the patient with these behaviors expects of the clinician-patient relationship.

The patient and family's perception, motivation, overt and covert priorities, and level of satisfaction are also ascertained. This can be accomplished through direct or indirect questioning, observations of behavior and attitudes, the patient's written daily calendar for medication and other therapies, and family assessment. Clinical experience and familiarity with the patient and family are valuable. Furthermore, asking the patient how he is feeling today and what he would like us to help him with has proved successful in identifying priorities, expectations, and enhancing satisfaction. At the completion of the visit, it is helpful to ask whether there are any questions, whether his priorities and needs have been met, and if the patient is satisfied.

Motivations become more apparent when the clinician and patient enter into negotiation about and goal setting for the regimen. The ability to contract a mutual agreement about the therapeutic plans and goals is affected by competing motives. Some motives the patient may identify; others are unconscious or covert. We have seen patients who temporarily undergo hypertension evaluation and therapy to acquire a desired job or other monetary benefits. Others undertake weight loss programs to appease partners' complaints. By ascertaining the patient and his family's life-style, one can begin to determine what his priority activities and the affecting variables are. To determine the consistency of the motivational level, the clinician can assess the patient's previous history and his perceptions of personal goal accomplishment. Ongoing evaluation and retrospective comparisons are important.

To determine the presence and level of patient resistance, hostility, and opposition (overt and covert), the clinician can assess appointment attendance and punctuality (lateness can reflect covert hostility). Previous and present medication and therapy adherence can be reviewed. Overt or openly expressed anger can be reflected in a situational context (e.g., "Rather than bother me with all these questions, just look at my chart."). Anger can also be carried over from other circumstances as in displacement or as a response to other internal processes such as grieving. An angry posture may be an inherent part of the individual's personality as in characterological anger. Covert anger and resistance can be expressed by frequent complaints about the health care rendered and strong attempts to control the clinician and treatment. Also those patients who demand considerable or extraordinary attention and care from the clinician may have covert anger.

Finally, both overt and covert forms of resistance and hostility can present or be provoked through unsatisfied mutual expectations, questions, and agreements.

The secondary measures of noncompliance, which involve the lack of modification of identified risk factors as jointly agreed on, are evaluated at each encounter. These are discussed in Chapter 6 and Appendix A. The remaining secondary parameter, the failure to demonstrate readiness to adhere to or accept the therapeutic regimen, is discussed earlier under the various considerations of the interactional parameters and in Chapter 6.

FACILITATING COMPLIANCE

Methods and strategies for facilitating compliance are incorporated through-out Chapters 6, 8, and 9. The suggestions are presented in capsulated form in this section.

The clinic environment and organization can be designed to promote com-pliance. This can be accomplished by demonstrating enthusiasm and commit-ment to high blood pressure control in the following ways:

1. Expand the staff's level of hypertension control knowledge and expertise.
2. Motivate staff to participate in and provide hypertension control services.
3. Prompt the staff to share their enthusiasm and concern about hyperten-sion with the patient population.
4. Ensure that all staff convey a consistent message to the population about hypertension.
5. Hold staff conferences routinely to discuss hypertension control services. Patient and family programs can be evaluated and new perspectives and approaches developed.
6. Encourage staff to elicit patient and family problems with compliance and to convey this information to the physician or nurse.
7. Place hypertension literature and posters in conspicuous and accessible locations.
8. Send hypertension literature and brochures to the entire clinic population, explaining the clinic's concern and commitment to hypertension control as well as the following:
   a. General blood pressure, cardiovascular risks, and hypertension infor-mation
   b. The importance of annual blood pressure checks for the entire family
   c. Routine blood pressure checks on all patients and their families as pro-vided by the clinic
9. Routinely measure blood pressure as part of all medical and nursing care.

An effective and accurate record and tracking system to monitor appointment attendance and medication needs to be maintained. Some functional approaches include the following:

1. Maintain a master file of elevated blood pressure screens and treated hypertensives. Minimize the time between an elevated blood pressure screening and the medical referral appointment.
2. Schedule appointments at close intervals until blood pressure control is achieved and generally not more than every 3 months thereafter.
3. It is essential that appointments be scheduled before the patient leaves the clinic and a written confirmation given. Try to accommodate to time and job conflicts and family problems.
4. Mail and telephone appointment reminders several days prior to the visit.
5. If the patient is unable to make an appointment, ascertain the reason and assist and accommodate accordingly.

6. Immediately telephone or mail clinic visit failure notices.
7. Check the medication supply and determine whether it is adequate until the new appointment.
8. Define and monitor the mechanism of follow-up and tracking of individuals who are repeated appointment failures.
9. Use a hypertension summary sheet for each individual.
10. Use a standardized interview, history, and educational summary form.
11. Collaborate with the pharmacist and write the patient's return visit date on the prescription.

To minimize patient inconvenience and secure continuity of care, the following procedures can be instituted:

1. Decrease waiting time.
   a. Schedule accordingly.
   b. Use paraprofessionals and clerical workers to perform the paperwork and measure basic parameters (blood pressure, height, weight, pulse).
   c. Send a hypertension questionnaire to new hypertensives prior to initial evaluation to facilitate data collection.
2. Conduct nurse entrance and exit interviews and/or possibly manage a case load of hypertensives.
3. Ensure that the patient is treated by the same clinician.
4. Order the minimal amount of laboratory and diagnostic studies necessary for appropriate evaluation.
5. Determine whether there are financial constraints and accommodate accordingly.

A highly individualized medication regimen that will promote compliance is essential. Steps that will facilitate this include the following:

1. Define the goals and time framework for the drug therapy. Provide feedback at each encounter regarding progression toward the goal.
2. Design a therapeutic regimen that is the easiest and least disruptive to the patient and family's preexisting behaviors, habits, and life-style.
3. Simplify the regimen.
   a. Use less tablets, less frequently.
   b. Use combination tablets.
4. Minimize the expense of the therapy.
   a. Whenever possible, use the least expensive brands and generic names.
   b. Initially and until dose titration stabilizes, order only the amounts of medication needed until the next visit and thereafter in economical quantities.
5. Anticipate and adjust for expected temporary adjustments and side effects from the drug therapy to allay patient anxiety and address patient concerns for therapeutic safety.
   a. Prior to initiating treatment, fully explain potential side effects with detailed instructions as to what the patient should do if they occur.

b. Differentiate between side effects and expected temporary adjustments to drug therapy. For example, diuretics will produce urinary frequency during the initial few weeks. After that time, the urine output returns to near prediuretic levels. The patient needs to know this to prevent interference with job activities or sleep and to dispel the notion that the medicine has "stopped working" when the urine output normalizes. Thiazide-induced alterations in serum potassium levels are presented differently. We inform the patient of his baseline potassium level, the normal ranges, and the mechanisms by which thiazides decrease serum potassium within the framework of expected changes. Adverse side effects occur when serum potassium levels drop below the stated normal range or symptoms (described fully) present.

c. Clear instructions as to what the patient should do if side effects or problems with drug therapy occur are necessary. We encourage our patients to call the clinic and discuss the problem with the involved staff. We discourage the practice of stopping the drug therapy or taking other medications. When expected temporary adjustments do occur, we frequently reassure the patient that his body and blood pressure need time to adjust to the new therapy and the clinic staff is available to discuss problems and alter plans as necessary.

6. Ascertain and clarify misperceptions. Discuss what the therapy is, why the medication is needed, how it works, what to expect, the adjustments the patient may expect, and the beneficial outcomes. Refer to the Veterans Cooperative Study findings, which demonstrated the efficacy of drug therapy in terms of lowering the numbers of cardiac, cerebrovascular, and renal complications. Perceptions regarding cardiovascular risk factor modification as one form of treatment of hypertension may be changed by referring to the Framingham study which first identified those risks and resultant complications. This can be conveyed through slides, posters, and graphs.

a. Focus the expectations and priorities of the different aspects of hypertension treatment.

b. Jointly define the priorities, goals, expectations, and prescribed activities as appropriate.

c. Close collaboration with open candid lines of communication with physician is essential. This unites the physician and nurse in a patient advocacy role. Other health professionals such as pharmacists, social workers, and dieticians are involved in varying degrees. However, in our setting the physician-nurse collaboration directs, interprets, and determines the therapeutic regimen through jointly negotiating goals, priorities, and health care activities with the patient and significant other. The amount, type, and method of health care delivery by allied health professionals need to be considered, since this may interfere with or confuse the patient's therapeutic focus and negotiated priorities. We have ongoing and frequent communication between health members coordinated by physician and nurse.

7. Incorporate family participation and supervision and utilize the health team approach. As the patient desires we encourage families and significant others to attend clinic and participate in the services and educational programs. Home visits may be beneficial to determine and facilitate compliance and retrieve nonattenders. Home blood pressure measurement is an excellent "control" tool for certain individuals and families. This tracking also provides the clinician with more representative blood pressure readings.

8. Label the medication bottles exactly.
   a. Write (or have the patient write) the instructions.
   b. Give the patient a medication brochure further explaining and reinforcing the necessity of taking the medication.
   c. Inform the patient when he is expected for a return visit, why, and what he can expect.

9. Suggest the use of a medication calendar, which can be brought and discussed at each visit. Encourage the patient to jot down feelings and circumstances on the medication calendar when taking the medications as well as problems with the drugs or adherence. Positive and negative patterns and influences begin to emerge which can be reinforced where appropriate and discouraged or considered for modification if detrimental. When the calendar is reviewed at each clinic visit, this reinforces the need, importance, and value of the drug therapy and adherent behavior.

10. Consider the variety of behavioral modification techniques and utilize the most desirable and appropriate. (Join medication behavior with a daily routine activity such as brushing the teeth or eating lunch.)
    a. Identify target behavior.
    b. Determine what environmental circumstances surround the experience (positive and negative).
    c. Jointly design therapeutic goals (short-term and long-range) including liberal support and encouragement for appropriate behavior and discouragement for noncompliance.

11. Consider using written patient contracts when they are mutually comfortable and appropriate. Clearly define through negotiation what the goal is, what the patient can expect from the health professional, and what is expected of him and the time framework. Evaluate progress and provide the rewards and reinforcement for success. For example, a patient may agree to take medications as prescribed for 3 months with no more than ten failures, based on medication calendars and blood pressure

levels. Consider prepaid commitment fees or other token rewards (when relevant and appropriate), which are returned (as reinforcements) to the patient when appropriate, clearly defined health behaviors or goals are accomplished. Discourage noncompliance. Renegotiate the contract as necessary.

12. Consider selective nonattention techniques. Spend less time with non-compliers and more time with compliers, providing reinforcement, attention, and support.

13. Emphasize and continuously reinforce the following:
    a. It is necessary to take medication every day.
    b. Do not stop or change doses of the medication without discussing this with the clinician.
    c. Do not take other medications without the clinician's knowledge and approval.
    d. Always call the clinician when not feeling well or experiencing side effects.

Considering and accommodating for psychologic factors that affect compliance may be necessary as follows:

1. Assess and support patient and family coping mechanisms. The healthy mechanisms and strengths can be supported and utilized to promote adherence. Other types of professional assistance may be indicated for the unhealthy coping mechanisms. Employ their coping mechanisms as a parameter of patient and family's ability and readiness to learn and assume responsibility for his care.

2. Clarify misperceptions and erroneous attitudes and beliefs by means of counseling and health education. Strategies fostering attitudinal change include films such as *The Silent Killer,* with actor Ben Gazzara viewing three hypertensive men and their progress; *The Hard Way,* with Bill Cosby attempting to increase black teenagers' awareness of hypertension and its relevance to them; *Getting Down on High Blood Pressure,* in which hypertensive blacks fully illustrate and discuss the disease and treatment; and *Understanding High Blood Pressure,* in which good animation personifies and simplifies the disease process and treatment. Approaches such as varying fear content in the health messages and persuasion can also be utilized to alter erroneous beliefs and perceptions.

3. Determine and reinforce appropriate perceptions and beliefs. Again utilize approaches such as positive feedback, recognition, and encouragement.

4. Promote confidence in the health care rendered and the prescribed regimens through positive conviction and tone.

5. Attempt to achieve high levels of patient and family satisfaction in the following ways:
    a. Address the patient and family's agenda priorities, perceptions, and

needs. Simply asking what the patient would like to discuss today and using open-ended sentences help in this regard.

  b. Provide reinforcement, feedback, encouragement, support, and information.

  c. Convey interest, friendliness, warmth, and an understanding of the patient and family's concerns (empathy).

  d. Communicate openly and honestly and convey a tone of acceptance and desire to answer questions. Listen and do not prejudge or assume.

  e. Utilize and reinforce the patient and family's strengths to enhance compliance.

  f. Convey pride and satisfaction with the patient and family's progress and accomplishments (however small).

  g. Share the progress with the patient and his family. This may include the hypertension summary sheet with the results and meaning of the physical examination and laboratory tests. Comparing the initial chest x-ray films with the subsequent x-ray films to demonstrate how treatment decreased the size of the heart is helpful. Comparing ECG and laboratory results with previous interpretations is another method. All parameters are compared to previous visits, "his range of normal" described, and variations explained.

6. Reflect on interactions with the patients. Increase self-awareness (attitudes, responses, gut feelings, motivations, priorities) and adjust accordingly.

7. Avoid a formal, disdaining, and overbearing posture.

8. Allow tension to be released during the interaction.

9. Avoid mutual attempts at controlling one another or major disagreements. Utilize the patient's active input.

10. Adjust authority levels to meet the autonomy and dependency needs of individual patients.

11. Utilize a comfortable level of approachability and avoid overt and covert distancing maneuvers. Respect the same on the patient's part.

12. Evaluate personal responses.

  a. Was there acceptance in the resistant behavior?

  b. Was there rejection of the resistant behavior?

  c. Were there feelings of anger and was that conveyed?

  d. What was the clinician's level of aggressiveness with therapy in terms of failing to increase dosages as a result of patient anxiety, obesity, direct opposition, or no specific causes?

  e. Were there reflexive responses to aggravating or irksome behavior?

SUMMARY

"Compliance" can be defined as maintenance of an assigned therapeutic regimen. "Noncompliance" is said to exist when a patient does not adhere to the prescribed therapeutic regimen. Noncompliance may occur through a variety of mechanisms and be manifested by behavior patterns such as delaying required medical care, avoiding preventive community programs (blood pressure screening), appointment and medication failures, and resisting and/or not maintaining the prescribed therapeutic regimen.

The magnitude of this problem in medical and nursing practice is considerable. In terms of noncompliance with hypertension treatment, approximately one third of patients take their medicine conscientiously, one third occasionally, and one third rarely.

There is no singular proven theoretical model for noncompliance. Inconclusive data have been extracted from sociologic and demographic considerations and psychologic factors. Patient factors such as feeling less vulnerable, less concerned with their health, less confident in the physician's diagnosis and the certainty of his decisions, and the perception that the disease is less severe have been found to affect compliance. Patient motivations, priorities, and their degree of control over health matters have been found to affect compliance significantly. Compliant behaviors need to be viewed by the patient as useful steps toward valued and relevant goals and more beneficial (time, effort, and cost) than other activities.

In terms of medication and therapeutic regimens, the regimen that is simplest, easiest, and least disruptive to preexisting behavior and life-style is adopted. Furthermore, minimizing duration, cost, dose size and frequency, and number of drugs taken does enhance compliance. Little data is available regarding side effects precipitating noncompliance.

Social and emotional support is necessary for compliance.

There is conflicting evidence as to how health education enhances the patient and family's ability to adhere to therapy. The degree of fear arousal inherent in the educational message elicits certain behavioral responses. Depending on the individual's perception and coping mechanisms, this can either affect compliance positively or negatively.

It has been found that clinicians overestimate adherence considerably. Actions that the clinicians undertake in cases in which noncompliance is suspected are detailed explanations, convincing credible appeals, threats, and case withdrawal. The clinician who conveys interest, friendliness, warmth, and an understanding of the patient's concerns has been found to increase patient satisfaction but not necessarily adherence. However, patients with high levels of satisfaction are more likely to comply.

An analysis of physician-patient interaction has yielded evidence that noncompliance can be attributed to difficult and disturbed communication such as a formal and disdaining physician attitude, failure to discharge tension, mutual attempts at controlling one another, and lack of agreement. The techniques through which clinicians prevent or dissuade patient communication or questions are conspicuous surveying of the clock and waiting room; indistinct or inarticulate murmuring; disregarding, stopping, or interrupting patient communication; telephone interruptions; and initiating the interaction by receiving a disease rather than a person. Other clinician behaviors that contribute to noncompliance are related to nonaggressive therapy. These include failure to increase medication dosage due to patient anxiety, definite patient opposition, and attributing the cause of the hypertension to obesity.

The monitoring of compliance can be incorporated into each clinic visit. Our measures are indirect and the cutoff point at which compliance stops and noncompliance begins is negotiable, since each patient and family is viewed and treated on an individual basis. In terms of facilitating compliance, designing the therapeutic environment and regimen that is simplest and least disruptive to the patient's life-style promotes compliance. Detailed consideration of the factors that influence and the outcomes of the clinician-patient interaction is necessary.

Any combination of appropriate strategies to facilitate compliance are applicable, depending on the patient, significant others, health professionals, clinical setting, and resources involved. Nursing research is vitally necessary in the area of compliance with therapeutic regimens. The responsibilities and contributions of nursing in this critical area need to be assumed and expanded more aggressively.

SUGGESTED READINGS

1. Becker, M. H., Drachman, R. H., and Kirscht, J. P.: Predicting mother's compliance with pediatric medical regimens, J. Pediatr. **81:**843-854, 1972.
2. Becker, M. H., Drachman, R. H., and Kirscht, J. P.: A new approach to explaining sick role behavior in low income populations, Am. J. Public Health **64:**205-216, 1974.
3. Bowden, C. L., and Burstein, A. G., Psychosocial bases of medical practice: an introduction to human behavior, Baltimore, 1974, Williams & Wilkins Co.
4. Bowen, R. G., Rich, R., and Schlotfeldt, R. M.: Effects of organized instruction for patients with the diagnosis of diabetes mellitus, Nurs. Res. **10:**151-159, 1961.
5. Caplan, R. D., Robinson, E. R., et al.: Adhering to medical regimens, Ann Arbor Institute for Social Research, Ann Arbor, 1976, The University of Michigan.
6. Caron, H. S., and Roth, H. P.: Patient's cooperation with a medical regimen: difficulties in identifying the noncooperator, J.A.M.A. **203:**922-926, 1968.
7. Caron, H. S., and Roth, H. P.: Objective assessment of cooperation with an ulcer diet: relation to antacid intake and to assigned physician, Am. J. Med. Sci. **261:**61-66, 1971.
8. Davis, M. S.: Physiologic, psychological and demographic factors in patient compliance with doctor's orders, Med. Care **6:**115-122, 1968.
9. Davis, M. S., Predicting noncompliant behavior, J. Health Soc. Behav. **8:**265-271, 1971.
10. Francis, V., Korsch, B. M., and Morris, M. J.: Gaps in doctor-patient communication, N. Engl. J. Med. **280:**535-540, 1969.
11. French, J. R. P., Jr., Kay, E., and Meyer, H. H.: Participation and the appraisal system, Hum. Relat. **19:**3-20, 1966.
12. Gillum R. F., and Barsky, A. J.: Diagnosis and management of patient noncompliance, J.A.M.A. **228:**1563-1567, 1974.
13. How to get patient compliance. In Dialogues in hypertension, vol. 2, No. 2, Philadelphia, 1975, Health Learning Systems, Inc.
14. Janis, I. L.: The contours of fear, New York, 1968, John Wiley & Sons.
15. Korsch, B. M., Gozzi, E. K., and Francis, V.: Gaps in doctor-patient communication. 1. Doctor v. patient interaction and patient satisfaction, J. Pediatr. **42:**855-871, 1968.

16. Podell, R. N.: Physicians guide to compliance in hypertension, West Point, Pa., 1975, Merck, Sharp & Dohme Co., Inc.
17. Sackett, D. L., and Haynes, R. B.: Compliance with therapeutic regimens, Baltimore, 1976, Johns Hopkins University Press.
18. Schoenberger, J. A., Stamler, J., Shekelle, K. B., and Shekelle, S.: Current status of hypertension control in an industrial population, J.A.M.A. **222:**559, 1972.
19. Stamler, J.: High blood pressure in the United States—an overview of the problem and challenge. In Proceedings of the National Conference on High Blood Pressure Education, Pub. No. (NIH) 73-486, Washington, D.C., 1973, National Heart and Lung Institute, U.S. Department of Health, Education, and Welfare.
20. Suchmann, E. A.: Preventative health behavior: a model for research on community health campaigns, J. Health Soc. Behav. **8:**197-209, 1967.
21. Wilber, J. A.: Detection and control of hypertensive disease in Georgia, U.S.A. In Stamler, J., Stamler, R., and Pullman, T. N., editors: The epidemiology of hypertension, New York, 1967, Grune & Stratton, Inc.

CHAPTER 8

Organization of a clinic for hypertension detection, treatment, and research

The need for a categorical approach to deal with the enormous problem of uncontrolled hypertension has become apparent. To meet this need, hypertension clinics have emerged throughout the country. The goals of these clinics include detection, evaluation, treatment, and follow-up of hypertensive patients. Most of these clinics are affiliated with hospitals, although some are associated with ambulatory care centers. Many internists interested in hypertension are initiating hypertension clinics in their offices. When a clinic is a part of community hypertension control program, one of its major functions is hypertension detection.

HYPERTENSION DETECTION

The blood pressure screening process described in this section is based on the recently published recommendations of the Joint National Committee on the Detection, Evaluation, and Treatment of High Blood Pressure.

The objectives of a hypertension detection program are as follows:

- To educate health care providers and consumers about hypertension
- To seek out opportunities for high blood pressure detection and control
- To conduct hypertension screenings
- To verify elevated blood pressure readings

• To refer and track the individuals with two confirmed elevated blood pressure readings to medical care for evaluation, diagnosis, treatment, and follow-up of hypertension

Education

Considerable progress has been made during the past five years in educating health care providers about hypertension control. The prevalence, existence of high risk populations, and the consequences of hypertension are now more widely recognized and accepted. The vehicles that have assisted with the dissemination of this information include an increased amount of literature about hypertension by medical and nursing professionals; continuing professional education programs; pharmaceutical firm publications; hypertension conferences, seminars and multidisciplinary symposia; nonprofit health organization assistance; radio and television media; and nursing and medical school curriculum changes focusing on hypertension control. However, more aggressive efforts specifically addressed at effectively implementing hypertension control programs in an identified community, motivating health care providers to work collaboratively with consumers to control hypertension, and maintaining hypertension control and compliance are needed. A greater understanding of the enormous problem of noncompliance with therapy to control hypertension is necessary. Recently, strategies to enhance compliance have been examined and recommended by various researchers. Additional strategies are needed that are more clearly defined and easily adaptable to patient, family, and community problems.

The public is now more aware of high blood pressure. However, the need for long-term control is not well recognized or accepted. Educating health care consumers about hypertension is indeed challenging. Suggested approaches include presentations at health fairs; family high blood pressure programs; radio and television media; presentations at local community-, school-, church-, or industry-sponsored activities; and posters at local supermarkets, shopping centers, and state or community fairs.

Depending on the specific ambulatory care center or private practice setting, the patient population can be reached and educated through variations of these approaches. Examples include mailing hypertension pamphlets to all patients, displaying a variety of hypertension education materials, holding group discussions, and having mini-presentations in the patient waiting areas.

Screening

Every available opportunity for hypertension detection should be sought and utilized.[11] High blood pressure detection cannot be done without education and follow-up components.[15] In addition to the mass screenings at public and private places, all individuals seen for medical-nursing care in all specialties and settings should have a blood pressure measurement at each encounter. Dentists and optometrists are other vital contributors to the detection of high blood pressure.

The procedures for measuring blood pressure during the screening process need to be clearly defined and reinforced with the screeners to ensure accuracy and uniform standards.

Initial blood pressure screening. The form used by the Milwaukee Blood Pressure Program for blood pressure screening is shown in the box on pp. 138 and 139.

Following is a detailed step-by-step description of the blood pressure screening process:

1. Have the person comfortably seated with arm clothing removed or positioned appropriately.
2. The individual can be thanked for being concerned enough to have his blood pressure checked.
3. Briefly explain what the blood pressure screening procedure is.
4. If a consent statement is required, obtain the appropriate signature after the written and oral explanations are provided. The explanations may include the assurance of confidentiality, release of liability, and permission to forward information to the designated physician.
5. After receiving the signature, complete the information in the first section (visit 1) of the screening form.
6. Measure the blood pressure and document accordingly.
7. Compare the blood pressure reading and the age to the designated screening criteria. If both the systolic and diastolic numbers are less than the criteria specified in that individual's age group, the blood pressure reading is normal.
8. This blood pressure reading is explained to the client by comparing his normal reading with the criteria for his age group. The reading is written on the client's hypertension brochure or pamphlet that is distributed during screening.
9. Provide counseling regarding the following:
   a. The definition of blood pressure and explanation of hypertension
   b. The prevalence and risks of high blood pressure
   c. Its silent but deadly nature
   d. The need for annual family blood pressure checks
10. If either the systolic or diastolic number is greater than or equal to the stated screening criteria for the client's age group, the blood pressure is elevated.
11. This is recorded in the appropriate section of the screening form and client's pamphlet. If an elevated reading is present and the client is not under treatment, the client may be provided with the following explanation:

> Your blood pressure reading today is _____. The blood pressure numbers that are the cutoff points which we use to ask people to return for another blood pressure check or to their doctor are _____ for your age. Your blood pressure is higher than that today, which may mean you are at risk for having hypertension. Your blood pressure needs to be rechecked within a week.

HYPERTENSION SCREENING FORM

ID No. _____ Phone No. _____ - _____

Name _____ _____ _____
      Last   First   Middle
                                                              initial

Visit 1

I authorize the Milwaukee Blood Pressure Program (MBP) to administer blood pressure related medical tests to me and, if referral to a physician is needed, to exchange blood pressure–related information with my physician (or with any physician to whom my physician may refer me). I agree to release MBP, its employees, and agents from any and all liability that might result from tests made by MBP.

_____ _____ / _____ / _____
Signature   Date

Street address

City or town   Zip code

Birth date _____ / _____ / _____
Sex   1. Male 2. Female
Race   1. White 2. Black 3. Indian 4. Oriental 5. Latin
Do you have a family doctor?   1. Yes 2. No
Do you have high blood pressure? (told by physician)   1. Yes 2. No
Are you on therapy for high blood pressure?   1. Yes 2. No

Age _____   BP 1 _____ / _____

HIGH BLOOD PRESSURE CRITERIA
Age 18-49 ≥ 140/90 mm. Hg
50 and up ≥ 160/95 mm. Hg

If high: Return site No. _____   Return date _____ / _____ / _____
                              or
        Will you be seeing your own doctor? 1. Yes 2. No

Visit 2

Site No. _____   Date _____ / _____ / _____

Age _____   BP 2 _____ / _____
If normal: Return site No. _____   Return date _____ / _____ / _____
If high: Go to HISTORY

Visit 3

Site No. _____   Date _____ / _____ / _____

Age _____   BP 3 _____ / _____
If high: Go to HISTORY

Urinalysis   ☐ not received

Specific gravity ☐ . ☐ ☐ ☐   pH ☐ . ☐

Protein	0neg	1+	2+	3++	4+++
Glucose	0neg	1+	2+	3++	4+++
Blood	0neg	1+	2+	3++	4+++

HYPERTENSION SCREENING FORM—cont'd

History

Family

High blood pressure?	1. Yes	2. No
Stroke?	1. Yes	2. No
Heart attack?	1. Yes	2. No
Kidney disease?	1. Yes	2. No

Patient

Heart disease?	1. Yes	2. No
Oral contraceptives?	1. Yes	2. No
Smoking?	1. Yes	2. No
Overweight?	1. Yes	2. No
Headaches?	1. Yes	2. No
Chest pain?	1. Yes	2. No
Palpitations?	1. Yes	2. No

Physician/clinic No. _____

Name _____

Address _____

City _____ Zip _____

Phone No. _____ - _____

Appointment ☐ made ☐ to be made AM

Date ____ / ____ / ____ Time ____ : ____ PM

Comments

12. A full explanation of blood pressure and hypertension, the prevalence and risks of high blood pressure, its silent but deadly nature, and the need for a blood pressure recheck can be given. Various motivational strategies may be employed, depending on the screener's assessment and ability and the client's responses and needs.

13. Arrange an appointment for a return blood pressure screening. The client may be assisted to determine a convenient time and location (if other screening sites are used). Record the appointment information on the client's brochure and reinforce accordingly. Also record that information in the "visit 1" box on the return site and date lines. If the client will be seeing his physician for the blood pressure recheck, that information is written at the bottom of the screening form (physician/clinic, appoint-

ment, and comments). The client can be assisted to make the physician appointment. If the client decides to make his own appointment later, he can be informed that he will receive a call or letter within 2 weeks verifying the physician's appointment. The results of the blood pressure screening can then be forwarded to the physician prior to the appointment. Outreach activities and motivational strategies can be employed if the client fails to appear at the follow-up visit.

14. If a urine examination is conducted as a part of the repeat blood pressure screening, request that the client bring the first morning urine specimen in the bottle provided. The bottle needs identification in terms of the client's name, number, return date, and the time with instructions. The health care professional can explain that since high blood pressure may be related to kidney problems, the urine is tested for protein, sugar, and blood. This information along with the blood pressure reading is sent to his physician.

15. If an individual has an elevated blood pressure reading and is currently receiving medical therapy for hypertension, he is informed of his blood pressure reading and it is written on a recheck card. He is advised to tell his physician about the reading. The blood pressure reading can also be sent to the designated physician. The client can return monthly or as the physician requests for monitoring of blood pressure between physician visits.

16. If the individual states that he is not taking the medications as prescribed, record that information and begin more extensive hypertension counseling. It is necessary to emphasize the need for medical management and the importance of continuing the medication. Ask the client to call his physician to discuss this and assist as necessary. The private physician's name and address is obtained for follow-up. Notation of this problem or other concerns can be written in the "comment" section.

Second and third blood pressure screenings. It is necessary to document two elevated blood pressure readings before referring an individual to a physician for evaluation of hypertension. The procedure for a repeat screening is as follows:

1. Proceed as described in the first six steps of the initial blood pressure screening procedure.
2. Perform a dipstick urinalysis if a specimen is available. Record results in the urinalysis section of the screening form.
3. If the blood pressure is within the normal range:
    a. Inform the client of blood pressure reading and complete visit 2 section.
    b. Reschedule for third blood pressure screening.
    c. Counsel accordingly, including a thorough explanation that a third blood pressure reading is necessary since the first was high and the second normal.

  d. Answer the client's questions, clarifying misperceptions and reinforcing the hypertension counseling information. Additional motivational approaches may be utilized as necessary to promote screening follow-up.

4. If either the second or third blood pressure screening is elevated:

  a. Inform the client of blood pressure reading and complete visit 2 or 3 boxes.

  b. Obtain appropriate medical history information and record in history section.

  c. Counsel.

  d. Answer any questions.

5. Refer client to medical care.

Depending on the health care or screening setting, a new screening form for each visit need not be processed. To facilitate computer entry and outreach activities the Milwaukee Blood Pressure Program does utilize new forms with the same identification number for the same client at each visit. However, if blood pressure screening is incorporated into the medical and nursing care rendered routinely, the form can remain with the chart.

Hypertension screening in a health care setting. The following guidelines suggested by the Joint National Committee on the Detection, Evaluation, and Treatment of High Blood Pressure are recommended for hypertension screening at a health care setting such as a physician's office, emergency room, or ambulatory care facility:

Age	Blood pressure	Recommended action
All adults	Diastolic levels 120 mm. Hg or higher	Prompt evaluation and treatment
All adults	160/95 mm. Hg or higher	Confirm blood pressure elevation within 1 month
Below 50 years of age	140/90-160/95 mm. Hg	Blood pressure check within 2 to 3 months
Age 50 or older	140/90-160/95 mm. Hg	Check within 6 to 9 months

In a private practice setting, institution, or ambulatory care clinic, the nurse can incorporate blood pressure screening as part of all medical and nursing care. If an elevated blood pressure reading is found, it can be recorded in the chart where convenient and easily recognized for follow-up. If the patient is being treated by the physician for health problems other than hypertension and the blood pressure level is not severely elevated, a profile of blood pressure readings is necessary prior to initiating therapy. Following the time suggestions just described, a blood pressure recheck can be scheduled as part of the next clinic visit or a separate nurse visit. Our experience has shown that less time (under 2 weeks) between blood pressure rechecks enhances compliance.

Suggestions for a simple filing system to track these individuals through the blood pressure screening process are as follows.

1. Segregate hypertension charts from the main body of charts.
2. Design a master list of the hypertensive population. Divide the master list into sections on screening and treatment. The form list on hypertension treatment may include information on pertinent history, laboratory and x-ray results, ECG and other data, therapeutic regimen, educational summary, family assessment, work setting (industrial nurse collaboration), compliance, date last seen, return clinic appointment, outreach measures, and identified problems. This need not be so extensive, depending on the actual clinic charting and summary forms.
3. A color-coded flagging system can be clipped on to a chart corner. Multicolored dots, different for each month, can be attached to the flags. For example, Mr. Jones is being treated by the physician for a peptic ulcer and has had one elevated blood pressure reading. He has been rescheduled to return in a month. Therefore a blue dot is attached to his chart, which indicates a return during the next month. After review of chart flags against the master list or return checklist, outreach activities consisting of telephone calls, letters, or both can be instituted for appointment failures. Notations can be made on the chart and master index.
4. Color coding the master index file rather than the charts is another alternative. Following is an example of the color-coding system that we have found successful:
   a. If the patient misses a screening, an attempt is made to contact the patient and the master file card is flagged blue.
   b. If there is no patient response in 2 weeks, a second letter is sent and telephone contact is attempted. The file card is flagged green.
   c. If after 2 weeks the patient has not responded, another letter is sent and telephone call attempted. The file card is tagged yellow.
   d. If there is no response after 2 weeks, the patient is considered lost to follow-up, and the card is tagged black. However, personalized letters are still sent every 3 months.
   e. Severely elevated blood pressure levels or abnormal laboratory values are flagged red. Letters and telephone calls are processed daily to weekly until the patient responds.

The problem of the noncompliant individual during screening can be discussed by the health team to determine causes and devise appropriate approaches. Frequently, in a private practice setting the patient and family are known in varying degrees to the health team. This knowledge can be used to evaluate the situation and plan strategies addressing the individual and family's needs.

A special consideration with the outreach and follow-up process is confidentiality. For example, when the University Student Hypertension Clinic telephones a student who is residing at his family residence, the health staff does not identify the call as originating from the health center but from a university office. If the patient must be contacted at his place of employment, the same approach is used.

Utilizing volunteers for hypertension screening.[15] Volunteers may be involved in all phases of a hypertension control program. Their skills, abilities, interests, backgrounds, and education can greatly enrich and enhance hypertension detection and treatment efforts. The National High Blood Pressure Program suggests various aspects of community hypertension control in which volunteers may be involved:

- Planning procedures
- Data collection
- Evaluating health resources
- Interagency coordination
- Education component development
- Volunteer recruitment
- Publicity planning and implementation
- Outreach efforts
- Developing and dispersing written publicity
- Target population meetings
- Large scale publicity events
- Radio and television programs
- Public exhibits and seminars

More specifically, volunteers are used at the detection sites for the following activities:

- Blood pressure measurement
- Disseminate information
- Referral
- Clerical work
- Child care services
- Transportation
- Facility and equipment maintenance
- Trafficking crowds

In terms of follow-up, volunteers are used for making telephone calls and mail processing, home visits, record keeping, and initiating medical referrals.

We include the request for volunteer support in our prescreening publicity efforts. Advertisements for volunteers, which consist of posters, flyers, newspaper (local and community) articles, and requests to voluntary agencies and organizations, schools and other institutions, are distributed 3 to 4 weeks prior to the intended project. The tone and style of publicity varies with the target volunteer group. Highly motivated and enthusiastic key people can be utilized for recruitment. Both the supplier approach and the direct approach for recruiting methods are put into service. The supplier approach utilizes student volunteer programs in the university as well as service clubs, unions, churches, and volunteer bureaus. The direct approach targets the volunteers directly, such as person to person, newsletters, and group presentations.

Volunteers are requested to contact the designated staff person at the screening program office. This individual has the responsibility of procuring volunteer information (name, address, phone, previous experience in blood pressure screening, hours and site availability, preference in training session times), coordinating volunteer tasks, assigning site coverage, and master scheduling. All office personnel are briefed regarding the volunteer recruitment process. However, any questions or problems beyond simple measures are the responsibility of the volunteer coordinator. Volunteers are recontacted for confirmation of training session times and blood pressure screening assignment.

The training for volunteers wishing to participate in screening consists of two 90-minute sessions conducted by nurses. The first session consists of lectures, question-and-answer time, training film and audio cassettes, individual and group practice in the measurement of blood pressure, and counseling simulations. In the second session, highlights of the first session are reviewed (training film, audio cassette, and group and individual practice). A certificate is awarded if the volunteer functions proficiently as determined by the competency evaluation parameters.

Additionally, the following guidelines have been implemented:
1. Volunteers are reoriented and evaluated by the staff at the time of the actual screening assignment. This consists of performing several blood pressure readings with a staff member using the double-ear stethoscope and being closely evaluated. In addition, other pertinent aspects of blood pressure measurement at the screening process are reviewed at this time. This is documented on the volunteer record.
2. The volunteer is seated in close proximity to the staff member for the purpose of monitoring and assistance. The volunteer screening forms are checked prior to the client leaving the screening site.
3. All questionable, difficult, and elevated readings are the responsibility of the staff member.

Our volunteer information packet contains a thorough explanation of blood pressure and hypertension, proper blood pressure measurement technique, detailed step-by-step explanations of the screening process, administrative guidelines, sample screening form, common errors in blood pressure measurement, and common client questions and answers with counseling information. Personal and written appreciation is extended after their participation. A master index of volunteers is maintained for future use and availability.

In a private practice setting, volunteers from the patient population such as nurses who are not currently employed and other retired individuals can be utilized to screen in the waiting areas or assist with the outreach activities. However, confidentiality is a serious concern, especially in a small community. In an institutional clinic or community ambulatory care center, the ladies auxiliary, students, or retired individuals can be tapped for volunteer services.

Referring hypertensives for medical care

The process of referral of hypertensives for medical care must be clearly delineated prior to initiating the screening process. To accomplish this, conferences and discussions with the clinic, private practice, or institutional physicians during the planning stages of the screening program are necessary.

For individuals found to have diastolic blood pressure of 120 mm. Hg or more, immediate referral is indicated. Depending on the practice situation, the following procedures are recommended:

Private practice	1. Contact physician. Schedule client immediately into next earliest office hours.
	2. Send individual directly to emergency room of nearest hospital where physician has attending privileges. Notify physician.
	3. Consult immediately with physician about other options.
Ambulatory care clinic settings	1. Notify physician on duty for the day and present findings to discuss options.
	2. Send directly to affiliated emergency area with which ambulatory care clinic has reciprocal arrangements.
	3. If nurse practitioners are present, immediate referral can be made. Evaluation and treatment can be instituted according to protocol.
	4. Schedule immediately into next earliest clinic physician hours.
	5. Send directly to emergency room of nearest hospital.
Institutional independent nurse-managed clinics	1. Initiate evaluation and treatment according to protocol.
	2. Refer findings to consulting physician immediately for alternatives.
	3. Send to institutional emergency room and confer with treating physician.

For those individuals whose blood pressure readings are elevated but who do not require prompt treatment, routine referral is recommended. Sources of medical care utilized for both the large scale community and clinic office screening include private physician of choice, group practice physicians, primary care centers, family health care centers, community health centers, industrial treatment programs, and university student health treatment centers.

Blood pressure screening is one point of entry into the health care system. The method of referral may need revision periodically, depending on clinic loads, community response, and available staff. The most important consideration is the coordination, communication, and follow-up of referrals, for which the nurse is in a strategic position.

HYPERTENSION TREATMENT SERVICES

Once a suspected hypertensive has been referred into medical care, it is essential for proper treatment that the patient's blood pressure always be recorded as accurately as possible.

Accurate measurement of blood pressure

The indirect method of blood pressure measurement using a mercury sphygmomanometer has stood the test of time. It reflects closely true blood pressure as measured by an intraarterial needle.[2]

Procedure. The following procedure is recommended for arm blood pressure measurement over the brachial artery[8]:

1. Seat the patient comfortably with the brachial artery at heart level, the forearm flexed, and the palm upward. The limb can be resting on a flat surface.
2. Palpate the brachial artery for stethoscope application and to appraise systolic pressure for the appropriate degree of cuff inflation.
3. Verify the meniscus level of the mercury manometer to be exactly at zero. The manometer should be vertical at eye level.
4. Select an appropriate sized cuff and apply smoothly and snugly, with the lower margin approximately 2½ cm. or 1 inch above the antecubital space. The middle of the rubber bladder encased by the cuff is positioned over the anterior or ventral aspect of the arm.
5. Place the stethoscope diaphragm firmly and flatly over the brachial artery.
6. Simultaneously palpate radial artery and inflate the cuff rapidly to at least 30 mm. Hg above the point at which the radial pulse disappears. We suggest a minimum 220 mm. Hg as a guide for the lowest inflation point in adults.
7. Deflate the cuff at a rate of 2 to 3 mm. Hg/sec.
8. The Korotkoff sounds are evaluated as follows:
   a. Systolic pressure is the initial phase or the first sharp, tapping sounds. The first two consecutive beats are considered to be the systolic determination.
   b. Diastolic pressure is the onset of phase V or the complete disappearance of sound.

The leg blood pressure is measured over the popliteal artery with the patient in the prone position (lying on the abdomen). The popliteal artery is palpated. A thigh bag is used, since it is approximately 6 cm. wider than the arm bag. The added width and length of the cuff allow for the extra girth of the thigh. The cuff must be applied in such a manner that it lies evenly over the posterior aspect of the midthigh. The diaphragm of the stethoscope is firmly applied over the artery in the popliteal fossa. It is important to recognize that the systolic pressure in the thigh is 10 to 40 mm. Hg higher than that in the arm and that the diastolic pressure corresponds closely to the arm readings. It therefore is extremely important that the blood pressure reading be clearly recorded as a thigh measurement. In patients who cannot be positioned prone, the knee may be limitedly flexed to allow placement of the stethoscope over the popliteal fossa.

Equipment.[8,9] The cuff consists of inflexible and nonexpandable material, which encases the inflatable bladder. The material should be without defects such as torn seams, holes, or worn thin areas, which alter the manner in which the bag fills the cuff during inflation, resulting in erroneous readings.

The fasteners, or friction patches, that secure the cuff in place need to be checked periodically and replaced as necessary. The inflatable bag consists of a distendable rubber material. It is important that the width and length of the bag correspond to the diameter of the patient's arm. The highest pressure exerted by the inflatable bag is transmitted through the tissues at the center of the bag. For example, on an arm of average size with a standard size cuff, the pressure exerted at the center of the bag is adequately transmitted through to the brachial artery. However, if the cuff is not wide or long enough, the pressure exerted at the center of the bag will not adequately penetrate to the brachial artery, resulting in an erroneously high reading. It has been therefore suggested that the width of the bag exceed the diameter of the limb by 20%. More simply, an appropriately sized cuff would be approximately two-thirds the length of the upper arm. In addition, the length of the bag would completely envelope the arm without overlapping. The standard size bag for the average adult is 12 to 14 cm. wide and 23 cm. long. For obese persons or a thigh measurement, the cuff is usually 14 to 20 cm. wide and 35 to 40 cm. long. Elevated blood pressure readings in obese persons are evaluated with an index of suspicion. If an appropriate size cuff is not available, a forearm blood pressure measurement may be done.

Mercury gravity and aneroid manometers are most commonly used for blood pressure measurement. At each blood pressure measurement by a mercury manometer, the top rim of the mercury meniscus must be precisely at the zero point when no pressure is applied. If the meniscus is either above or below zero point, erroneous readings can result. Caution can be exercised so that the manometer is vertical and the meniscus positioned at eye level. The manometer tube must be free of oxidation, cracks, or missing numbers. The air vent must be cleaned, since obstructions may slow the responsiveness of the mercury column to bulb pressures. Loss of mercury should be avoided. This is a particularly hazardous concern in pediatric settings.

The tubing and rubber hand bulb can be inspected for cracks, porous areas, and loose connections. Particular attention to the area on the bulb where the fingers grip is necessary, since nails can wear and eventually perforate the rubber. The hand bulb then needs replacement.

The rubber tubing attached to the connecting joints can split, especially if different size cuffs are being interchanged. That area of the tubing can be cut back several inches and reconnected or replaced. Metal connecting joints or plastic adaptors made for use on other medical equipment should not replace defective connecting joints on blood pressure equipment. An adequate supply of parts needs to be kept available for the maintenance of blood pressure equipment.

To determine whether there is improper airflow through the system, the cuff can be rolled in the nurse's hand tightly, evenly, and snugly, or the cuff can be wrapped around a cylindrical solid object about the size of an arm, gripped firmly, and the system inflated and deflated.[9] During inflation and deflation, the responsiveness of the mercury up and down the column to the pressure changes can be observed. If too rapid a response is noted, the system is tested for the presence of an air leak. This can be accomplished by inflating the system to 250 mm. Hg or higher, then deflating to 200 mm. Hg and closing the air valve tightly. The pressure will be maintained at 200 mm. Hg if there is no air leak. If the loss of pressure is greater than 1 mm. Hg/sec., the tubing can be pinched firmly at 1-inch consecutive points from the manometer downward toward the hand pump. A leak would be reflected by a pressure drop between the compressed area and the manometer. Most commonly, air leaks are due to defective connecting joints; tears, holes, or porous areas in rubber tubing or bladder; or a defective air control valve. Defective parts need to be promptly replaced.

On the other hand, if the mercury column responds slowly or in a delayed fashion to the pressure changes, the pores of the kidskin diaphragm in the cap on the top of the mercury column may be blocked. Also, the mecury may bounce or will not elevate easily with a sealed valve. When this occurs, the cap on the top of the mercury glass column is unscrewed and the kidskin diaphragm replaced. If not available, some authorities recommend rolling the defective diaphragm through the fingers to open pores. However, we have found this not to be successful as a temporary repair measure. Another reason for a slowed mercury response can be an obstructed filter in the hand bulb or air valve. The tubing can be disconnected. The bulb and air valve are disassembled and the hand pump pressed several times to unblock the valve. In certain instruments with screen filters, cleaning or replacement of the filter is necessary.

The meniscus of the mercury can be checked by standing the manometer on an even flat surface. At eye level, the meniscus has a distinct, slightly rounded, and even line. A distorted meniscus may be due to dust or other matter in the mercury or along the glass column or the presence of bubbles. To empty the mercury, the cap is removed at the top of the glass column, and while gently tilting the top of the manometer up and down, the mercury is allowed to flow out into a clean, dry receptacle. If the mercury must be cleaned, it can be decanted slowly into a sheet of paper that has been rolled into a conical shape and placed in a clean receptacle. The opening at the peak of the cone is the size of a pin; thus the dirt and mercury oxide will be filtered out as it rises to the top of the fluid. The last few drops remaining in the filter paper are disposed of.

To clean the interior of the glass column, the glass column is removed, and pipe cleaners, detergent, or water is used to clean it. A final rinse with alcohol accelerates drying time.

Depending on the instrument, the reservoir can be cleaned as described earlier, or while still disconnected from the glass column and mercury fluid, the hand bulb can be pumped vigorously several times to blow dust out of the reservoir.

The glass column can then be reconnected with the manometer vertical on a flat surface, and the mercury can be replaced through a funnel or a paper cone. The meniscus can be calibrated and if greater than zero, the excess can be poured off. If less than zero, additional mercury can be inserted with a medicine dropper.

Between calibrations, a maximum limit of 5 mm. Hg/100 mm. Hg variation can be temporarily tolerated. How often a mercury manometer is checked and cleaned depends on the age of equipment, rate of use, and the condition. A minimum of once a year is required for cleaning and monthly for checking. In our clinic, the equipment is checked monthly, cleaned semiannually, and replaced annually.

Aneroid manometers are sensitive instruments that require careful handling. They can be recalibrated or repaired by the manufacturer or authorized agents. Once a month the aneroid instrument needs to be checked against an extremely accurate mercury manometer through a "Y" connector. The system is inflated to 250 mm. Hg and the pressure released. Halting the deflation at 5- to 10-point intervals over the entire range and comparing the two readings determine the accuracy of the aneroid. If the difference exceeds ±4 mm. Hg, the aneroid is not accurately calibrated. Aneroid manometers operate through metal bellows, which become elongated as pressure increases. The gear components transfer this action to the indicator needle. Some aneroid instruments have stop pins that counteract needle oscillation. Therefore incorrect calibration, which is usually perceived by altered needle positioning especially at the zero mark on deflation, may not be seen. An aneroid manometer without stop pins is accurate to ±3 mm. Hg when the indicator needle returns to zero on complete deflation. An important consideration is that mishandling this piece of equipment can produce inaccuracies that are not discernable at zero but exist at other points.

Two types of blood pressure equipment have been recently marketed. The random zero sphygmomanometer (Hawksley) is a conventional 0 to 300 mm. Hg instrument. However, it is fitted with a zero shifting device and constant airflow discharge valve. The zero level is randomized between 0 to 60 mm. Hg by a cam altering the mercury level in the reservoir. The true zero is determined after the usual blood pressure measurement is performed. The difference between the zero and random zero is subtracted from the systolic and diastolic levels. This reduces the effect of observer prejudice in blood pressure measurement. We utilize this piece of equipment in hypertension research projects.

There are other new automated devices such as the Audiometric 100 (Bodimetric Profiles), which electronically transmits and magnifies the sounds in registering system. An audible reading (without the use of a stethoscope) is then determined. The problems with this instrument concern calibration and detection of inaccuracies.

Other automated digital devices have been developed for consumer use and charge a fee for usage. These have been installed in shopping centers and pharmacies. The computerized Vita-Stat device generally provides an accurate reading. However, the machine must be checked and calibrated routinely to ensure accuracy. The drawback of screening by computers is that well-informed health professionals are not present to recheck the reading, provide counseling, or refer appropriately.

Finally, new types of equipment for home blood pressure measurement have become available. Generally, the problem involves poor construction, and the person is not able to determine errors or calibrate. In addition, some new blood pressure cuffs have the stethoscope permanently attached to the lower rim. This enhances convenience but may reduce accuracy and proper sound transmission.

Korotkoff sounds.[14] The tapping sounds and murmurs heard over an artery distal to a deflating blood pressure cuff are called "Korotkoff sounds." The name is derived from a Russian physician who in 1905 characterized the sounds and separated them into three phases as auscultated during indirect blood pressure measurement. The sounds were subsequently divided further into the five phases now utilized. The phases are differentiated by the qualities of the tapping sounds and whether a murmur is present (Table 4).[14]

The recording of systolic pressure is clearly delineated as phase I, or the initial sharp tapping sound. Two consecutive beats are auscultated. If by palpation the systolic pressure is higher than by auscultation, it is recorded as such.

The definition of "diastolic" blood pressure is controversial.[8] The American Heart Association in 1967 recommended that diastolic pressure be considered the onset of muffling, or phase IV. Some of the reasons include the physics of the transmission of sound in the circulation, which considers velocity, turbulence, vortices of flow, and the pressure gradients within altered channel diameters. Other reasons included the experimental results that phase IV fluctuates less than phase V after exercise, activity, and other increased cardiac output states such as thyrotoxicosis, severe anemia, and aortic regurgitation. In the presence of these conditions, in children who have been postulated to have a higher velocity of flow, and in other persons with a suspected hyperkinetic circulation, phase V may not appear, and sounds are audible down to the zero point.

Conversely, Maxwell and others[11] purport that phase V or the disappearance of sound is closest to true diastolic pressure. His experience as well as that of others indicate that among observers the recording of phase V corresponds more closely in range than the recording of phase IV. To avoid variations in blood pressure readings between observers, phase V is taken as the patient's diastolic blood pressure. Furthermore, certain individuals lack phase IV, and most physicians now recognize diastolic pressure as the disappearance of sound. The actual judgment as to precisely when the absence of sound begins is contingent on the extraneous noise levels, the hearing acuity of the observer, and the placement

Table 4. Korotkoff sounds

Phases	Character of sound	Physiologic processes
Phase I	Faint sounds appear. Later they intensify in clarity and pitch to distinct tapping.	Cuff pressure exerted on artery exceeds intraarterial systolic pressure and collapses artery. As cuff pressure is decreased, peak of systolic pulse wave is greater than applied cuff pressure, and blood surges into artery. Sharpness of tapping depends on forcefulness, speed, and quantity of surge of blood. Pulse does not appear initially because of inadequate quantity of blood distal to cuff. As cuff pressure lessens, more blood passes through radial artery and pulse is ascertainable.
Phase II	At onset of second phase, tap is followed by murmur. Tapping becomes progressively less audible and murmur more apparent.	As constricted artery dilates, countercurrents reverberate blood and blood vessel walls, creating murmurs. In average adult, phase II starts 10 to 15 mm. Hg after initial sounds of first phase and continues for 14 to 20 mm. Hg.
Phase III	Murmurs disappear. Tapping sounds become louder and higher pitched	Constricted artery continues to dilate as cuff pressure subsides. Systolic pulsations from heart maintain widened caliber of artery but during late diastole, artery narrows.
Phase IV	Tapping sounds suddenly become lower in pitch. Muffling appears.	Pressure exerted by cuff is less than intraarterial diastolic pressure.
Phase V	Absence of sounds; silence.	Normal caliber of artery is reestablished.

and condition of the stethoscope. Ravin[14] suggests that the onset of the fifth phase is somewhat less than the true diastolic pressure and the onset of phase IV is 4 to 8 mm. Hg higher.

On the basis of these controversial considerations, the World Health Organization, American Heart Association, and other authorities recommend recording both the onset of phase IV and phase V in the following manner: 120/76/68. This will more clearly delineate and relate figures to clinicians who may determine either phase IV or V to be the criterion for the diastolic pressure. This is also important for individuals who have a phase IV measurement 10 to 15 mm. Hg greater than phase V (e.g., 164/96/78). In this case, we consider the phase IV reading as the diastolic level.

The "auscultatory gap" is the diminution of audible sounds which can occur toward the end of phase I and through phase II. The sounds reappear during the third phase. This can present a serious problem, since the gap may span a 40 mm. Hg difference, and the systolic pressure erroneously may be determined as too low. To avoid this mistake, the artery to be compressed by the cuff can be palpated as the cuff is rapidly inflated to at least 30 mm. Hg above the point at which the pulse disappears. In addition, we utilize a minimum of 220 mm. Hg as a guide for the lowest inflation point in adults if pain is not present, since the vasospasm in response to the pain can alter the blood pressure.

If cuff inflation is slow, congestion of the blood vessels can result, producing an auscultatory gap. If no murmur is audible or the pulse pressure is low, an auscultatory gap is suspected. The procedures that amplify Korotkoff sounds are described on the opposite page.

Clinical implications of variations in Korotkoff sounds.[14] *Pulse pressure* can be obtained by subtracting the diastolic pressure from the systolic pressure, which is normally one third of the systolic pressure. High pulse pressure may be due to systolic elevations as a result of arteriosclerosis, a high cardiac output state, or a decreased diastolic blood pressure as in aortic regurgitation. A reduced pulse pressure may be attributed to low cardiac output states such as shock, pulmonary embolism, or obstruction such as aortic stenosis.

Irregular cardiac rhythms can render inaccurate blood pressure determinations. This is related to fluctuating stroke volume and therefore blood pressure from one cardiac cycle to another. The previous pulse cycle and stroke volume specifically affect the systolic pressure. On the other hand, the pulse pressure has an inverse relationship to the length of the pulse cycle. This means that an extended pulse cycle due to an altered cardiac rhythm lowers the diastolic pressure of that cycle and elevates the systolic pressure of the next one.

In *atrial fibrillation* due to the irregular heart beat and pulse variation, blood pressure determination is difficult. A sequence of blood pressure readings can be performed and averaged. The "systolic level" is defined as the average pressure at which the greatest number of beats are audible.

There are differences in blood pressure during the *respiratory cycle*. Normally these differences are an elevation during expiration and a decrease on inspiration. These differences reflect alterations in the vascular capacity of the lung tissue due to the intrapleural pressure variations during the respiratory cycle. In constrictive pericarditis this difference may be more dramatic and the accompanying pulse abnormality is called "pulsus paradoxus." To observe the difference during the respiratory cycle, the cuff can be deflated slowly around the systolic range. Varying lengths of silent periods between beats will be heard.

Conditions affecting blood pressure measurement.[12] Sources of error that render blood pressure determinations inaccurate are as follows. The *position* the patient assumes during blood pressure measurement is a common problem. He must be comfortably seated for at least 5 minutes with the arm on a flat surface at level of the heart (fourth intercostal space). With the brachial artery above

PROCEDURES TO AMPLIFY KOROTKOFF SOUNDS

Techniques	Physiologic basis
Elevate the patient's limb above heart level prior to cuff inflation. This enhances venous return. Inflation is then performed with the limb elevated.	Circulation to the limb distal to the cuff is temporarily occluded during inflation. The pressure of the blood in these vessels depends on the quantity of blood trapped and the capacity of the vascular bed. A smaller quantity of blood in a larger capacity vascular blood bed lowers the forearm pressure. This increases the pressure differential of the blood surging through the compressed artery to the distal vessels, intensifying the tappings and murmurs. Elevating the limb prior to cuff inflation therefore decreases the quantity of blood distal to the cuff, amplifying the sounds.
Quickly inflate the cuff while palpating the distal artery to a point 30 mm. Hg higher than the point of disappearance of the pulse.	As the cuff is inflated, the venous return is occluded first. Slow inflation traps blood distal to the cuff with each pulsation. Quick inflation lessens the quantity of blood distal to the cuff, amplifying the sounds.
Lower the arm and instruct the person to open and close his hand quickly eight to ten times.	The muscular exercise expands blood vessels and their capacity, decreasing the pressure in the limb distal to cuff.
Deflate the cuff at a relatively rapid rate of 2 to 3 mm. Hg/sec.	Slower inflation produces congestion in the venous vessels distal to the cuff and elevates the diastolic level.
Let the cuff deflation proceed completely to zero.	Halting deflation between the systolic and diastolic levels and again inflating the cuff to ausculate for systolic pressure refills the distal blood vessels and alters the sounds. A minimum of 2 minutes should therefore elapse before another reading is attempted.

this level, the blood pressure readings will be erroneously low. Conversely, if the brachial artery is lower, the blood pressure readings will be higher. This is due to the differences in the hydrostatic pressure.

Postural changes such as moving to a supine position can also alter readings; thus the measurement can be performed 5 minutes after the patient assumes the supine position. Usually the arm is close enough to the heart level so that alterations in position are not required. If postural hypotension is being evaluated, blood pressure should be measured 2 minutes after standing.

The sphygmomanometer need not be at heart level; however, it does need to be at eye level.

A *loose cuff* causes elevated systolic and diastolic levels due to the bloating of the middle of the inflatable bag, which minimizes the width efficiency, mimicking the problem of a narrow cuff. If the stethoscope is applied too firmly, murmurs can be created or sounds may be audible down to the zero point. The stethoscope should never be placed under the rim of the cuff, since inappropriate pressures will be exerted on the stethoscope, which alters the reading. Also the stethoscope *tubing* should be freely suspended and not in contact with any material or surface that can cause extraneous sounds. Extraneous sounds in the immediate surroundings may interfere with proper auscultation or make the patient uncomfortable or apprehensive. This is especially true of a busy outpatient clinic, hospital ward, or emergency room. Every attempt needs to be made to control environmental stimuli.

Observer abilities such as hearing, concentration, and response time affect auscultation. Since the Korotkoff sounds are low frequency, generally around the hearing threshold range through a stethoscope, the hearing ability of the observer is crucial. There may be varying degrees of hearing loss, which can be either congenital in nature or acquired. The observer or treating clinician may not be cognizant of this loss. Based on this concern, blood pressure measurement training programs should include some type of auditory testing. The teaching stethoscope, which has two ear sets, may be somewhat helpful in this regard.

Variations in observer concentration and response time can produce significant differences in blood pressure readings. This is difficult to evaluate. Frequent rest periods during continuous blood pressure recording sessions are mandatory. Frequently, in a fatigued state, one can confuse auditory and visual cues. Response time can also be affected by painful stethoscope ear sets and aching hands from frequent pumping of the hand bulb.

The *observer's preconceived ideas,* either conscious or subconscious, in terms of overreading or underreading a blood pressure measurement may be present. This may be especially true when the observer is either overcommitted or noncommitted to detecting hypertension. This happens with newly trained observers more frequently. Adequate prescreening training and education minimize this. To check these screeners, their screening forms can be identified in some manner (code, numbers, letters) and examined periodically.

It has been well documented that some observers demonstrate a predilection for the numbers "zero" and "five." Strong emphasis that blood pressure readings are determined to the nearest even number is necessary.

Blood pressure measurement in children.[17] A National Task Force report on blood pressure control in children released in April 1977 has detailed the guidelines for the appropriate methodology and instrumentation of blood pressure measurement in infants and children. The emphasis is that repeated blood pressure measurements over a period of time rather than a single or isolated reading are essential for consistent and meaningful observations. Interpretation of blood pressure measurements in children differs from that in the adult as a result of the following circumstances:

1. Different arm sizes require a correspondingly appropriate cuff.
2. In infants, the Korotkoff sounds generally are not audible due to their low sound frequency.
3. Blood pressure measurement in anxious, active, and restless children is difficult to perform.
4. Blood pressure is labile especially in adolescents.
5. Distortions and errors in auscultation of Korotkoff sounds can occur with heavy stethoscope pressure on the antecubital fossa.
6. Phase IV of the Korotkoff sounds is considered to be the measure of diastolic pressure.

Appropriate cuff size (inner inflatable bladder) is imperative for obtaining accurate readings. The following dimensions are recommended:

	Bladder dimensions (cm)	
Cuff name	**Width**	**Length**
Newborn	2.5-4.0	5.0-10.0
Infant	6.0-8.0	12.0-13.5
Child	9.0-10.0	17.0-22.5
Adult	12.0-13.0	22.0-23.5
Large adult arm	15.5	30.0
Adult thigh	18.0	36.0

The inflatable bladder needs to completely envelope the arm without overlapping. By using the largest cuff that will fit snugly rather than using the one with the appropriate cuff name (newborn, infant, etc.), fewer errors will be encountered.

The environment and conditions under which the child will have a blood pressure measurement must be conducive to support, comfort, and reassurance.[7] This is critical for the child under the age of 10 years whose ability to fantasize and perceive this procedure as painful and/or intrusive is extremely active. For this age group, conditions can be manipulated to assist the child to relax, promote a rapport with the health staff, and explain simply what will be done. Children under 6 years of age may feel most secure and relaxed sitting in their mother's lap. Infants are usually supine, being quieted with a bottle or a pacifier. In conjunction with a physical examination, vaccination, injection, or any other type of anxiety-producing procedure the blood pressure reading can be obtained prior to the procedure. It is well known that the anxious, apprehensive, crying child may elevate his systolic pressure 20 to 50 mm. Hg.

The auscultatory technique in infants is inaccurate because the sounds are too faint. The two methods that can be employed are the Doppler and flush techniques. The Doppler method uses an electronic instrument that interprets the different levels of sound of the blood movement into discernable frequencies. The systolic determination is considered to be accurate; however, the diastolic accuracy has not been well documented. The flush method generally applies to infants under 1 year of age and is as follows. Elevate the arm about heart level. The area of the midforearm to the fingers is wrapped with an elastic bandage. The cuff is applied proximal to the bandage. Lower the extremity and quickly inflate the cuff to 30 mm. Hg above the disappearance of the radial pulse. Remove the bandage rapidly and slowly proceed with cuff deflation. The final point of determination is the first manifestations of the flush, which is the mean blood pressure and recorded as such. Blood pressure measurements in children over the age of 3 years should be performed and plotted annually on a percentile curves chart as provided in the National Task Force report.

Clinic procedures

An orientation pamphlet describing the clinic procedures is helpful and can be issued at the time the initial appointment is made.

Depending on the setting, the scheduling of hypertensive patients can be accomplished in various ways. In our clinic, the nurse performs the history in about 30 minutes. Either the nurse or clinical assistant can obtain the physical parameters of height, weight, body frame estimation, pulse, and blood pressure in both arms sitting and in one arm standing. We follow and treat according to the arm with the highest blood pressure measurement at rest. Another 15 to 30 minutes is allotted for a physical examination by the physician. The therapeutic alternatives and plans are then discussed in detail with the patient. The patient then returns to the same nurse for an exit interview. This consists of additional counseling, interpreting therapeutic regimens, support, and scheduling the next appointment. This usually takes 5 to 20 minutes.

In an independent nurse–managed clinic, the nurse can perform all the aforementioned activities, including evaluation and initiation of therapy, according to the protocol. On a regular basis, cases are reviewed with the responsible physician.

Role of paramedical personnel. Paramedical personnel can be utilized effectively in a hypertension clinic or private practice setting. Their primary responsibilities include measuring the physical parameters, obtaining specimen samples for laboratory work, performing ECGs, reinforcing hypertension counseling, promoting compliance, and performing clerical work. Prior to the initial clinic visit, our paramedical personnel perform the following duties:

1. Mail reminder letters during the week preceeding the scheduled appointment.
2. Telephone patients the day prior to the scheduled visit for a confirmation. The patient or family's response is noted on the chart. If the patient cannot keep the appointment, all attempts are made to determine the reason. The appointment time is rescheduled to suit the patient's convenience.

3. Assemble all charts for the upcoming week. This process includes the following:
   a. Inserting needed chart sheets
   b. Transferring summary data to the new sheets
   c. Identifying all chart data
   d. Updating laboratory data
   e. Pulling master file cards to verify current resident and telephone number at the time of the visit
   f. Inserting identified computer sheet in chart

After the scheduled clinic, the charts are reviewed jointly by the physician and nurse and the documentation process is completed.

After an extensive orientation, continuing education for the paraprofessionals includes weekly staff meetings and monthly in-service sessions. Both professionals and paraprofessionals identify educational interests and needs. After considering these and related factors such as identified problem areas, new information, theories or techniques, and hypertension education materials, the nurse can circulate an outline of the topic for the upcoming in-service session a week prior to the intended date. This includes an invitation for further suggestions and revisions. The in-service presentations are evaluated by the staff and revised accordingly.

For additional staff development in an ambulatory care clinic or private practice setting, steps that the nurse can take to educate and motivate health staff about hypertension control include imparting genuine enthusiasm and concern about hypertension control; explaining and clarifying the needs and benefits of quality hypertension control; and incorporating the staff in the planning and organization of the hypertension control activities. This includes jointly defining the goals for hypertension control for the population and unique setting, delegating responsibility for the development and implementation of various components of hypertension control, and assigning the responsibility for groups of patients to individual staff members.[13]

Other educational approaches include the following[6]:

• Procuring and making easily available to staff resources for learning about hypertension control
• Identifying oneself as a flexible resource or facilitator who can direct the staff to appropriate resources
• Utilizing in-service sessions, group discussions, patient-staff teaching sessions, self-instruction learning program tools, clinical conferences, audiovisual materials, and other activities as methods of teaching

Role of the nurse practitioner.[10,16] The nurse's role can be divided into four categories: patient care management, education, clinic supervision, and research.[6,10]

Patient care management. The nurse's activities include organizing and providing high-quality hypertension detection services for a variety of community settings and groups, facilitating and tracking the entry of suspected hypertensive individuals into the health care system, and orienting the hypertensive patient and family to hypertensive disease, treatment, and control. The nurse manages a stable hypertensive patient population in the following ways:

1. Assessing health status and cardiovascular risk profiles through pertinent history, physical examination, and relevant laboratory or other tests
2. Interpreting the information obtained and considering alternate actions as defined by the clinic protocol or physician directives
3. Prescribing or adjusting medications and therapy according to protocol standards and patient collaboration and negotiation
4. Providing thorough explanations of the medical-nursing care to the involved patient and family and eliciting their participation
5. Evaluating and revising prescribed therapy according to protocol specifications and other appropriate parameters
6. Initiating, coordinating, and monitoring patient referrals and resource use as necessary
7. Consulting and collaborating with the physician in the following manner:
   a. Reviewing and discussing each patient case prior to and after the nurse clinic visit
   b. Documenting patient care activities appropriately
   c. Consulting with physician as warranted
8. Identifying, managing, and monitoring patient and family compliance with medical-nursing regimens
9. Diagnosing, managing, and evaluating nursing problems through the formulation, application, and evaluation of nursing care plans (independence-versus-dependence conflicts, body image disturbances, environmental problems, psychologic adaptation to chronic illness)
10. Evaluating the delivery and outcomes of patient care through quality assurance programs and periodic audit and revision

Education. The nurse's role is to organize, plan, implement, and evaluate hypertension education and counseling services during the detection phase of hypertension control for both screeners and clients. In addition the nurse can provide education and risk factor modification services to identified hypertensive individuals and their respective families as follows:

1. Assess patient learning needs and abilities.
2. Design and plan appropriate teaching goals, strategies, and methods.
3. Implement individualized hypertension education and risk factor modification programs.
4. Evaluate and revise the programs periodically.

Additional nursing activities may be to seek out and review various and new hypertension educational approaches, materials, and methods; furnish in-service education, training, and development to the hypertension clinic and screening staff; provide continuing education services to nurses practicing in a variety of health care settings; teach undergraduate and graduate nursing students the theoretical and clinical applications of hypertension control; and engage in educational activities and coordinate the hypertension control services of various community service groups.

Clinic supervision. The nurse's supervising activities may be as follows:

1. Utilizing appropriately available administrative, organizational, and human resources to facilitate, support, and maintain high-quality hypertension control activities
2. Promoting, designing, implementing, and evaluating nursing practice and hypertension control innovations
3. Promoting an effective communication network
4. Supervising and evaluating subordinates effectively to enhance growth and development and to improve the delivery of patient care services

Clinical and epidemiologic research. The nurse's functions include planning and investigating specific problems related to hypertension control. The nurse also assists the physician in designing and implementing protocols to investigate new antihypertensive agents and collects data for epidemiologic research. One can continually review the pertinent literature for advances in hypertension control as well as assist and interact with other agencies interested in conducting research with the clinic patient population. In addition, the nurse can develop and participate in other hypertension control investigations and present research findings at appropriate scientific meetings as well as publish.

All research protocols must be first approved by a human research committee.

Joint practice relationship[11]

The joint physician-nurse practice relationship is highly individualized.[3] Considering the legal parameters, interactional levels, and the independent, dependent, and interdependent functions, there is no set "recipe" for a successful joint practice. However, several components of the physician-nurse joint practice relationship strongly influence its success. Depending on one's particular situation, the following discussion may be helpful.

The first component is mutual respect and trust, which is a significant part of the foundation of the relationship. This develops with time and experience. In considering the independent, dependent, and interdependent role functioning, there is great variation in each clinical setting and among individuals. In addition, the limits and constraints in one setting may be different than in others. With experience, both individuals become more comfortable with these levels of functions and limits. For example, when a problem or complication arises that exceeds the nurse's protocol and independent role limits and a physician is not present, she can attempt a telephone consultation or have access to another physician. The physician's confidence and trust in the nurse's judgment and her recognition of one's limits are crucial. Furthermore, the nurse needs to have reciprocal confidence and trust in the physician's support of her reasonable actions. Verbal orders can represent a serious problem in this respect if trust and confidence are lacking.

The manner in which the physician approaches patient needs and their required actions differs from that of the nurse.[11] The physician traditionally reacts to a disease state by assimilating all relevant data, evaluating and diagnosing a condition, and prescribing the appropriate therapeutic interventions. This scientific method is based on knowledge, training, and sophistication acquired during medical school and clinical experience. The nurse solves patient care problems by employing the nursing process, whereby she performs a comprehensive assessment of patient and his family's biologic, psychologic, and social needs. The nurse shares this information with the physician and utilizes this data to develop a composite picture of patient and family needs. Rather than delineate one or two diagnoses, the nurse jointly determines and negotiates the priorities and manner in which the patient and family needs are satisfied. Certain needs will be satisfied by the physician's contributions, some by the nurse, and others through appropriate resources and referral. The individualized objectives and goals for the delivery of health care to a patient and family and their required actions are then jointly defined between physician, nurse, and patient and family. This relationship is ongoing and the evaluation and revision must be continuing.

In a hypertension clinic, the nurse primarily manages stable hypertensives and develops and coordinates various facets of hypertension control services. The physician cares for the severe and uncontrolled hypertensives with or without complications and other acute or episodic illnesses. These functions may overlap or vary, depending on the patient and family's needs or problems.

Collaborative decision making in a joint practice, as discussed earlier, involves mutual respect, trust, and maturity. Both professionals must focus on "our patient" as opposed to "my patient." Of course there will be disagreements, but the determination and respect necessary to make a successful joint venture in quality patient care will temper them.

The subsequent managerial responsibility for patient care again is variable. The first important point is that the patient understand that the care received is jointly provided, that the physician and nurse as a team provide health care to meet their needs. Second, irrespective of who is the current manager of a particular patient's care or whether the patient is being seen in the physician clinic or nurse clinic, the joint relationship must continue with agreement about the care provided.

The ultimate responsibility for the health care rendered is with the physician. In this regard, the following actions are suggested:

1. All laboratory reports and other data are reviewed and signed by the nurse. Charts are reviewed prior to and after each clinic visit. The abnormal laboratory, x-ray, or other relevant data are brought to the physician's attention. Physician's directions regarding abnormal laboratory, x-ray, or other data are recorded in the chart. Telephone conversations with patients are also notated on the chart.

2. During the chart review, the alternatives are discussed and agreement

reached. It is essential that the nurse clearly understand and record those agreed plans. The physician notes referrals and consultations in the patient's records. Prescriptions are signed by the physician. Our mechanism for controlled substances is that the physician signs the prescription for the designated patient, which is then valid for a 24-hour period. If the patient misses his appointment, the prescription is destroyed.

3. The protocol must clearly designate which problems are outside the realm of the nurse's practice and the mechanism defined for physician consultation.
4. Patients may elect to see the physician at their discretion.
5. In-depth, comprehensive, accurate, and legible medical records need to be maintained.
6. The physician's countersignature is required on all records.

In terms of the *legal aspects concerning the use of protocols,* there is no clear definition.[1,5] A protocol is a written tool delineating for the clinician the methodologic and sequential collection of data and the subsequent appropriate alternatives and actions. If the data is correctly collected, the stated sequence of deductive logic leads to accurate and exact decision making. The protocol must be validated, medically accepted, evaluated, and revised periodically. The parallelism of protocols to standing orders is intriguing but not defined as yet. The exact legal interpretation of protocols employed as part of a joint practice endeavor is unclear at this time.

It is understandable that the physician feels uneasy about relinquishing some degree of control and supervision of patient care activities. With the expansion of the nurse's role and responsibilities, many states have revised their definitions of nursing and nursing functions. Most notable are the revisions in the areas of diagnosis, treatment, and independent nursing functions. The nurse can consult state, local, and institutional laws to acquire a definite understanding of her status and function.

Fee structures in a joint practice vary. The fee for the initial visit is higher because of greater time spent by both the physician and the nurse. The fee for the return visit with a physician is higher than a visit in the nurse clinic. Generally, in most ambulatory settings, the patient pays a single fee to the physician or institution. The nurse receives a set income. However, the physician's income varies with numbers of patients, types of medical services, and other factors. In some solo or group practice facilities, the nurse practitioner shares the profits on a sliding scale. For example, the nurse may receive 25% of the fees received on the patients she manages.

DATA PROCESSING AND EPIDEMIOLOGIC RESEARCH IN HYPERTENSION

With hypertension control emerging as a national priority in health care, there is a pressing need for further epidemiologic research in hypertension control. The Veterans Administration cooperative study, the National Hypertension Detection and Follow-up Program (NHDFP), and the Community Hypertension Evaluation Clinic (CHEC) Program are some examples of well-coordinated projects that have provided much useful information on hypertension and its control.

Use of computers

Computers have revolutionized our ability to store and analyze data. The computer not only performs calculations, but it assists and augments trained cerebral activity. It is the responsibility of health professionals, particularly those interested in research, to familiarize themselves with the fundamentals of computer operation and work closely with computer programmers and statisticians to facilitate advancement of knowledge. Blind opposition, blind acceptance, or abdication of responsibility to computer experts can cause great harm.

A computer programmer programs the computer on the basis of knowledge and experience acquired by individuals at the peak of their competence in a given field. The knowledge is then preserved in the computer. Later, a neophyte can draw on this body of knowledge simply by pressing a few buttons. This is the basic advantage of the use of computers.

Collection of hypertension screening data. For proper collection of data, it is necessary to use appropriately designed forms. The forms developed by the Milwaukee Blood Pressure Program for hypertension screening are shown on the following pages. The completed forms are transported to a computer terminal and the information entered in the computer for storage and analysis.

Data collection for patient management. Two forms have been developed for collection of pertinent data regarding management of patients in our hypertension clinic. The form shown in Fig. 9 is used for the initial evaluation. Its design is based on the history and physical forms discussed in Chapter 4. It can be easily adapted to various needs.

The form used for transmitting follow-up information is shown in Fig. 10. A separate form is used for each visit. The information is later entered in a computer for storage and further analysis. At regular intervals, usually once a year, a computer printout is obtained for each patient summarizing all the follow-up information.

Additional printouts are obtained at 3- to 6-month intervals which provide information on the total clinic population and various segments based on age, sex, race, and other factors. Also blood pressure control, weight, smoking habits, alcohol consumption, medications, side effects, and other variables are analyzed. This information is helpful in the evaluation of hypertension and risk factor control, medication side effects, and the occurrence of hypertensive complications among the clinic population.

Confidentiality of medical records. With the use of computers, the retrieval of information is rather easy. The health information shared by an individual at the time of screening or developed at the time of evaluation is always confiden-

Text continued on p. 169.

INITIAL VISIT INFORMATION

HP1   01
1 3   4-5

IDENTIFICATION

Patient No. [   ]   Date [   ]   Age [   ]
         6   11   Mo.   Day   Year   18   19
                                              12   17

Race 20 [   ]   1. White 2. Black 3. Indian 4. Spanish 5. Asian 6. Other

Sex 21 [   ]   1. Male 2. Female   Place of residence   [   ]
                                             (census tract)   22   25

Mode of
referral   [   ]   1. Directly from walk-in clinic
             26   2. Downtown Medical and Health Services screenings
                                3. Milwaukee Blood Pressure Program screening other
                                   than Downtown Medical and Health Services
                                4. Other physician
                                5. Self-referral
                                6. Milwaukee County Medical Complex
                                7. Other

HISTORY

Previously informed   [   ]   Previously treated   [   ]   1. No
of hypertension   27   for hypertension   28   2. Yes, but dis-
                                                                            continued
                                                                         3. Presently on
                                                                            treatment

Symptoms

Asymptomatic   29 [   ]   Occipital or morning headache   30 [   ]

Epistaxis   31 [   ]   Cardiac symptoms   32 [   ]

Vascular symptoms   33 [   ]   Cerebrovascular symptoms   34 [   ]

Renal and   35 [   ]   Pheo   36 [   ]   Aldo   37 [   ]
urinary tract   symptoms   symptoms
symptoms

Smoking   [   ]   1. Nonsmoker   Alcohol   [   ]   1. None or
           38   2. Less than 1 pack/day   39   occasional
                           3. 1-2 packs/day   2. Weekends
                           4. >2 packs/day   3. Daily ($\leq$2
                                                                           drinks/day)
                                                                        4. Alcoholic

Birth control pill   [   ]   1. Never
or estrogen   40   2. In the past
                                   3. Presently on pill or estrogen

Fig. 9. Sample form used to transmit the initial patient visit information for computer storage.

Continued.

PHYSICAL EXAMINATION

Weight [ ] 41
1. Normal
2. <20% overweight
3. ≥20% overweight

Actual weight [ ] 42 44

Blood pressure [ ] 45
1. Normal
2. Mild hypertension
3. Moderate hypertension
4. Severe hypertension

Blood pressure reading [/] 46 48 49 51

Signs of cardiac decompensation [ ] 52
1. None
2. S₄ present
3. Other signs

Signs of retinal-vascular disease [ ] 53
0. Normal
1. Grade I/IV
2. Grade II/IV
3. Grade III/IV
4. Grade IV/IV

Signs of peripheral vascular disease [ ] 54
1. Carotid
2. Peripheral
3. Carotid and peripheral

LABORATORY RESULTS

Urine [ ] 55
1. Normal
2. Protein
3. Glucose
4. Blood
5. Protein and glucose
6. Protein and blood
7. Granular casts
8. RBC casts
9. Protein and casts
10. Protein, blood, and casts

Hematocrit [ ] 56
1. Normal (40-45)
2. High (>45)
3. Low (<40)

F.B.S. [ ] 57
1. ≤110
2. >110

BUN (creatinine) [ ] 58
1. <20 (<1.5)
2. 20-40 (1.5-3)
3. >40 (>3)

Serum potassium [ ] 59
1. >3.5
2. 3-3.5
3. <3

Serum cholesterol [ ] 60
1. ≤200
2. 201-300
3. >300

Serum triglycerides [ ] 61
1. ≤200
2. 201-300
3. >300

Serum uric acid [ ] 62
1. <10
2. ≥10

Serum calcium [ ] 63
1. ≤10.5
2. >10.5

SGOT [ ] 64
1. <40
2. 40-60
3. >60

Peripheral renin [ ] 65
1. Low
2. Normal
3. High

Chest x-ray [ ] 66
1. Not done
2. Normal
3. Enlarged heart
4. Incidental findings
5. Enlarged heart and incidental findings

IVP [ ] 67
1. Not done
2. Normal
3. Suggestive of reno-vascular hypertension
4. Other abnormalities

Fig. 9, cont'd. For legend see p. 163.

LABORATORY RESULTS—cont'd

ECG ☐ 68   1. Not done
              2. Normal
              3. Left ventricular hypertrophy
                 (LVH)
              4. Ischemia
              5. LVH and ischemia
              6. Myocardial infarction
              7. Other changes

Other tests ☐ 69   1. Not done
                     2. Normal
                     3. Abnormal

ASSESSMENT

Diagnosis ☐ 70   1. Normotensive
                   2. Labile hypertension
                   3. Essential hypertension
                   4. Secondary hypertension

Associated conditions   Obesity ☐ 71   Diabetes ☐ 72   Gout ☐ 73

Hyperlipidemia ☐ 74

Complications of hypertension   None ☐ 75   Cardiac ☐ 76   Cerebro-vascular ☐ 77

Retinal ☐ 78   Vascular ☐ 79   Renal ☐ 80

Significant incidental findings   ☐ 81   1. None detected
                                            2. Detected

TREATMENT

None ☐ 82   Diet alone ☐ 83   Weight loss ☐ 84

Behavior modification ☐ 85   Diuretic ☐ 86   Propranolol ☐ 87

Methyldopa ☐ 88   Reserpine ☐ 89   Clonidine ☐ 90

Prazosin ☐ 91   Hydralazine ☐ 92   Guanethidine ☐ 93

Other drugs ☐ 94

Fig. 9, cont'd. For legend see p. 163.

FOLLOW-UP VISIT INFORMATION

HP2 Follow-up visit sequence No. [   ] (enter 2 or higher)
1 3   4   5

IDENTIFICATION

Patient No. [   ]   Date [   ]
            6   11   Mo. Day Year
                                          12   17

HISTORY

Return appointment   [   ] 1. As scheduled
                         18   2. <1 month late
                                  3. ≥1 month late
                                  4. Transferred to another physician
                                  5. Moved
                                  6. Lost to follow-up
                                  7. Discharged
                                  8. Died

Symptoms

Asymptomatic   19 [   ]   Occipital or morning headache 20 [   ]

Epistaxis   21 [   ]   Cardiac symptoms   22 [   ]

Vascular symptoms   23 [   ]   Cerebrovascular symptoms   24 [   ]

Renal and urinary   25 [   ]   Pheo symptoms   26 [   ]
  tract symptoms

Aldo symptoms   27 [   ]

Smoking   [   ]   1. Nonsmoker
              28   2. <1 pack/day
                         3. 1-2 packs/day
                         4. >2 packs/day

Alcohol   [   ]   1. None or occasional
              29   2. Weekends
                         3. Daily (≤2 drinks)
                         4. Alcoholic

Medications [   ]   1. Taken as directed
              30   2. Irregular in taking medication
                         3. Discontinued

Fig. 10. Sample form used to transmit the follow-up patient visit information for computer storage.

HISTORY—cont'd

Side effects

None   31 ☐   Symptomatic postural 32 ☐
                                            hypotension

Sexual inadequacy   33 ☐   Allergic reaction   34 ☐

Hypokalemia   35 ☐   Gout/hyperuricemia   36 ☐

Diabetes/hyperglycemia   37 ☐   Tiredness/lethargy   38 ☐

Nasal congestion   39 ☐   Other   40 ☐

PHYSICAL EXAMINATION

Weight   ☐ 1. Normal   Actual weight ☐
           41   2. <20% overweight   42   44
                 3. ≥20% overweight

Blood pressure   ☐ 1. Normal   Blood   ☐   /   ☐
              45   2. Mild hypertension   pressure 46 48 49 51
                    3. Moderate hypertension reading
                    4. Severe hypertension

Signs of cardiac   ☐ 1. None   Signs of retinal-   ☐
decompensation   52   2. S₄ present   vascular disease   53
                       3. Other signs   0. Normal
                                              1. Grade I/IV
                                              2. Grade II/IV
                                              3. Grade III/IV
                                              4. Grade IV/V

Signs of peripheral vascular disease   ☐ 1. Carotid
                                     54   2. Peripheral
                                          3. Carotid and peripheral

LABORATORY RESULTS

Urine   ☐ 1. Normal   6. Protein and blood
      55   2. Protein   7. Granular casts
            3. Glucose   8. RBC casts
            4. Blood   9. Protein casts
            5. Protein and glucose   10. Protein, blood, and casts

Hematocrit ☐ 1. Normal (40-45)   F.B.S.   ☐ 1. ≤110
         56   2. High (>45)   57   2. >110
               3. Low (<40)

BUN   ☐ 1. <20 (<1.5)   Serum potassium ☐ 1. >3.5
(creatinine) 58 2. 20-40 (1.5-3)   59   2. 3-3.5
               3. >40 (>3)   3. <3

Continued.

Fig. 10, cont'd. For legend see opposite page.

LABORATORY RESULTS—cont'd

Serum cholesterol 60 ☐
1. ≤200
2. 201-300
3. >300

Serum triglycerides 61 ☐
1. ≤200
2. 201-300
3. >300

Serum uric acid 62 ☐
1. <10
2. ≥10

Serum calcium 63 ☐
1. ≤10.5
2. >10.5

SGOT 64 ☐
1. <40
2. 40-60
3. >60

Peripheral renin 65 ☐
1. Low
2. Normal
3. High

Chest x-ray 66 ☐
1. Not done
2. Normal
3. Enlarged heart
4. Incidental findings
5. Enlarged heart and incidental findings

IVP 67 ☐
1. Not done
2. Normal
3. Suggestive of renovascular hypertension
4. Other abnormalities

ECG 68 ☐
1. Not done
2. Normal
3. LVH
4. Ischemia
5. LVH and ischemia
6. Myocardial infarction
7. Other changes

Other tests 69 ☐
1. Not done
2. Normal
3. Abnormal

ASSESSMENT

Diagnosis 70 ☐
1. Normotensive
2. Labile hypertension
3. Essential hypertension
4. Secondary hypertension

Associated conditions   Obesity ☐ 71   Diabetes ☐ 72   Gout ☐ 73

Hyperlipidemia ☐ 74

Complications of hypertension   None ☐ 75   Cardiac ☐ 76   Cerebro-vascular ☐ 77

Retinal ☐ 78   Vascular ☐ 79   Renal ☐ 80

Significant incidental findings ☐ 81
1. None detected
2. Detected

Fig. 10, cont'd. For legend see p. 166.

TREATMENT

None [____]
82

Diet alone [____]
83

Weight loss [____]
84

Behavior modification [____]
85

Diuretic [____]
86

Propranolol [____]
87

Methyldopa [____]
88

Reserpine [____]
89

Clonidine [____]
90

Prazosin [____]
91

Hydralazine [____]
92

Guanethidine [____]
93

Other drugs [____]
94

Fig. 10, cont'd. For legend see p. 166.

tial. Only personnel involved in the patient's care should have access to it. It should under no circumstances be given to a third party without the patient's express written consent. Whenever the information is used for epidemiologic research, the patient's identity is never revealed. The confidentiality of the medical records cannot be overemphasized.

Directions for future research

Hypertension screening and control programs offer an excellent opportunity to perform useful epidemiologic and clinical research. In the following sections, a few of the areas in hypertension control that await answers are discussed.

Factors predisposing to hypertension. Stress, high-salt intake, excessive alcohol consumption, heredity, obesity, and drug abuse are believed to predispose to hypertension. Why these factors lead to hypertension in certain individuals and not in others is not clear.

Pathogenesis of essential hypertension. The cause of essential hypertension remains obscure. Several mechanisms have been proposed to explain its pathogenesis. Most investigators have their favorite hypotheses. Further research is urgently needed to clarify how these mechanisms operate in relation to one another.

Antihypertensive therapy. The role of behavioral modification as the sole therapy for hypertension is controversial. Which technique of relaxation and what life-style changes are most effective in lowering blood pressure are questions that remain unanswered.

New and better drugs are needed that would lower blood pressure without the side effects of present medications. It is unlikely that a drug will be discovered that will "cure" essential hypertension, but it may be possible to develop effective therapeutic agents that need to be taken only once a week or once a month. With the development of such an agent, the problem of patient noncompliance may be dramatically changed.

•   •   •

These and many other aspects of hypertension need further research. Systematic collection of data and appropriate analysis is likely to prove helpful in solving some of the outstanding questions.

SUMMARY

Hypertension clinics have emerged throughout the country for detection and treatment of hypertension. The process of hypertension detection includes professional and public education, hypertension screening, verification of elevated blood pressure, and referral of suspected hypertensives. Volunteers can be effectively utilized in the various phases of a hypertension control program.

For proper treatment of hypertension, it is essential that blood pressure be recorded as accurately as possible. The mercury sphygmomanometer is probably the most reliable instrument for this purpose. Regular maintenance of equipment is necessary for adequate performance.

The sounds produced by the movement of blood across a narrowed artery are called the "Korotkoff sounds." Phase I of the sounds corresponds with the systolic blood pressure and the phase V with the diastolic blood pressure. Conditions that can lead to errors in recording of blood pressure include position of the patient, defective equipment, and observer errors.

For diagnosis of hypertension in children, repeated blood pressure measurements tracked over a period of time rather than a single or isolated reading are essential.

Paramedical personnel can be utilized effectively in a hypertension clinic for measuring the physical parameters, performing clerical work, and promoting compliance by reinforcing hypertension counseling. The nurse's role includes patient care management, patient-family education, clinic supervision, and research.

Several components of the physician-nurse joint practice relationship influence its success. These include mutual respect and trust, recognition of one's limits, sharing of responsibilities, proper utilization of the protocol, and the physician's support of the nurse's reasonable actions.

Hypertension control can be effectively accomplished in a variety of health care settings with minimal disruption of usual services and routines. The different components of the detection and treatment phases of hypertension control can be varied to meet the needs of a given clinical situation.

A pressing need for further research in the epidemiology, pathophysiology, treatment of, and nursing contributions in hypertension control exists. Computers are a great help in storage and analysis of data. It is the responsibility of health professionals to familiarize themselves with the basics of computer operation. For proper collection of data, it is necessary to use appropriately designed forms. The confidentiality of medical records should be protected at all costs.

SUGGESTED READINGS

1. Bullough, B.: The law and the expanded nursing role, New York, 1975, Appleton-Century-Crofts.
2. Burch, G. E., and DePausquale, N. P.: Primer of clinical measurement of blood pressure, St. Louis, 1962, The C. V. Mosby Co.
3. Capell, P. T., and Case, P. B.: Ambulatory care manual for nurse practitioners, Philadelphia, 1976, J. B. Lippincott Co.
4. Carter, L., and others: Standards of nursing care: a guide for evaluation, New York, 1976, Springer Publishing Co.
5. Creighton, H.: Law every nurse should know, Philadelphia, 1975, W. B. Saunders Co.
6. Ganong, J. M., and Ganong, W. L.: Nursing management, Germantown, Md., 1976, Aspen Systems Corp.
7. Greenfield, D., and others: Children can have high blood pressure too, Am. J. Nurs. **79:**770-772, 1976.
8. Kirkindall, W., and others: Recommendations for human blood pressure determination, New York, 1967, American Heart Association.
9. Lancour, J.: How to avoid pitfalls in measuring blood pressure, Am. J. Nurs. **79:**773-775, 1976.
10. Lewis, E. P.: The clinical nurse specialist, New York, 1970, American Journal of Nursing Co.
11. Mauksch, I., and Young, P.: Nurse-physician interaction in a family medical care center, Nurs. Outlook **22:**113-119, 1974.
12. Maxwell, M.: A functional approach to screening in the hypertension handbook, West Point, Pa., 1974, Merck, Sharp & Dohme.
13. Quality control and performance appraisal, vols. 1 and 2: a reader consisting of eight articles from the Journal of Nursing Administration Editorial Staff, 1976.
14. Ravin, A.: The clinical significance of the sound of Korotkoff (audiocassette), West Point, Pa., 1974, Merck, Sharp & Dohme.
15. United States Department of Health, Education, and Welfare: Handbook for improving high blood pressure control in the community, Washington, D.C., 1974, National High Blood Pressure Education Program.
16. United States Department of Health, Education, and Welfare: Guidelines for educating nurses in high blood pressure control, DHEW No. (NIH) 77-1241, Washington, D.C., 1977, U.S. Government Printing Office.

CHAPTER 9

Hypertension control at the work setting

OVERVIEW OF THE CHALLENGE

Within the past decade, new approaches to hypertension control have been successfully attempted such as utilizing the industrial or work setting.[1-3] From previous chapters, the epidemiologic facts regarding the problem of hypertension dramatically and clearly demonstrate the challenge to health care professionals. To more aggressively address this problem, the concept of worksite hypertension screening and treatment has evolved. The key to successful detection and long-term management of the estimated 30 to 50 million Americans having hypertension is cooperation between the public and private sector: between industry, government, health professions, and community organizations. The work setting is well suited for facilitating their cooperation.[4]

Several major studies have documented the prevalence and significance of hypertension in the industrial population. Schoenberger[6] found that approximately 20% of individuals in an industrial group have hypertension, 60% of which were undetected and untreated. The cumulative Milwaukee Blood Pressure Program data are presented in Figs. 1 and 2. Within certain work settings, we found a somewhat higher prevalence of hypertension—nearly 30%.

High blood pressure is an expensive killer. Industries have a large stake in this problem. Over 75 million Americans are employed of which 25 million may be hypertensives who, unaware of their problem, risk premature death and disability from a progressive disease that can be controlled.

The economic costs are astronomical.[4] The total economic cost of cardiovascular disease in the United States as estimated by the American Heart Association in 1976 was in excess of $20 billion of which almost $10 billion represent lost wages. Besides the lost income and cost of medical care, over 52 million work days of production a year were lost. Costs such as losses in management skills, labor turnover, personnel training and development, and production are difficult to calculate but staggering. For every employee killed by an industrial accident or disease, 50 die from cardiovascular disease.[6] The Social Security Administration ranks hypertension and its consequences as the largest single cause of disability in this nation. What is not included in the figures is the incalculable human toll resulting from premature death and disability.

The following discussion of hypertension control at the work setting is adapted from the relevant educational materials of the National High Blood Pressure Education Program.[4]

USEFULNESS OF INDUSTRIAL SETTING FOR HYPERTENSION CONTROL

Certain innate features in the worksite facilitate high blood pressure programs as follows:
1. The population is established and relatively stationary, which is important for follow-up procedures.
2. Reaching the population is easier.
3. Avenues for communication already exist.
4. Health care services are usually available on site and administered by a registered nurse and physician on either a full- or part-time basis.
5. Consolidated groups are present that by means of peer influence enhance compliance.
6. Physical facilities are available.

Benefits to employers

The benefits of an industrial hypertension control program to the employer are many and important to appreciate:
1. Absenteeism due to illness, physician visits, and hospitalizations is decreased.
2. The number of employees who would become disabled or the loss of productive employees is lessened.
3. Cost benefit advantages are not clearly delineated at the present time. Unfortunately, there is no distinctly reliable cost benefit study. However, the prevention of catastrophic illnesses such as cerebrovascular accidents or congestive heart failure through high blood pressure detection and con-

trol should definitely lead to a diminution of medical costs. Therefore health and life insurance rates as a fringe benefit paid by employers for the employees will be reduced. Also employers will be better able to determine the dimensions and productivity of their work force.

If a local community hypertension control program exists, the additional benefits derived from an industry cooperating with the local program include a faster and more efficient screening process; cost saving through free screening, staff, and supplies; and an outreach program to ensure follow-up of suspected hypertensives.

Benefits to employees

The benefits to employees include the following:
1. Complications of and the mortality due to hypertension are reduced.
2. A hypertension detection and control facility is readily available.
3. Awareness concerning the need for preventive health care and detection of high blood pressure is increased.
4. The financial benefits of hypertension detection and possibly treatment may be shared with the employer.
5. Hypertension detection and control services are received in an environment conducive to long-term compliance.
6. The employee is relating to one familiar health care team at the worksite for the detection and possibly management of high blood pressure.
7. There is cooperation between the industrial nurse and the private physicians. Services may include blood pressure monitoring, hypertension education programs, and renewal of the antihypertensive prescriptions between private physician visits.
8. The employee may receive hypertension counseling through the teaching modalities of individual and group sessions and written and audiovisual aides provided by the industrial nurse.

HYPERTENSIVES IN THE WORK FORCE

An important consideration for hypertensives in the work force is that of *employability*. Studies have revealed that identifying individuals as hypertensive may result in employment or promotion rejection.[7] The extent of this practice is difficult to determine. Utilizing this criteria in determining employability and promotion appears to have little relation to modern concepts in hypertension control. A more enlightened practice is one of nondiscrimination for employees with adequately controlled hypertension. With untreated individuals, aggressive attempts are necessary to motivate and educate. Suggestions to address the problem of confidentiality and job security may include having union officials and other employee representatives present during the screening programs. Management, however, would not be present.

In situations in which the employee's medical condition warrants protection from an occupational health hazard, the company physician may find confidentiality difficult. The medical evaluation may need to be interpreted or released with employee permission in workmen's compensation claims, absence, and assignment change or promotion. Boards of reviewing physicians may be made available for the prospective or present employees when a controversial situation arises. Furthermore, in terms of employability it is understandable that the cost of medical, life, and disability insurance to the employer is lessened if known uncontrolled hypertensives are not employed.[7]

Public safety with particularly *hazardous occupations* is another concern. Job situations in which the side effects of drugs might result in harm to the patient or others need to be avoided. For example, the FAA in consultation with the American College of Cardiology dictates that hypertensive pilots may fly if the blood pressure is controlled with appropriate medication and in the absence of target organ complications. Blood pressure measurement is required on a 3-month basis. The U.S. Department of Transportation has revealed recent statistics which indicate that more accidents than previously realized occur as a result of hypertension and other cardiovascular conditions. Consequently, appropriate blood pressure levels have been delineated for employed truck drivers.

WORKSITE HYPERTENSION CONTROL PROGRAM

The type and extent of an industry's hypertension control program depends on the population size and distribution of employees, the accessibility of company medical staff and services, and the commitment of both labor and management to address the problem.[5]

The following guidelines provide a comprehensive approach for a hypertension control system in industry. The suggested steps identified as necessary for the successful organization and implementation of such a program can be readily adapted and individualized for a particular company's needs. Excerpts from the experiences of the Milwaukee Blood Pressure Program in this area are interspersed throughout.

The fundamental elements for a hypertension control program at worksite are prescreening publicity and education, scheduled screening programs, referral process to medical care, follow-up of employees with elevated blood pressure, hypertension education program, and monitoring and treatment services for diagnosed hypertensives (optional).

Prescreening education and publicity

Prior to initiating a successful blood pressure screening program, the awareness level of the target industrial population can be increased relative to what hypertension is, its prevalence and complications, and the need for periodic blood pressure checks. In Chapter 6 a thorough explanation of this education process was presented. The difference is the vehicles used for employee exposure and the process of disseminating that information. Also, when initially presenting the prescreening publicity, utilizing the term "high blood pressure" instead of hypertension will avoid misinterpretation of the disorder as a nervous condition or emotional instability.

The vehicles for dissemination of information include the following:

1. High blood pressure posters strategically placed on bulletin boards and display facilities in the cafeteria, locker rooms, health clinic, and other locations
2. Company magazine and employee union newsletter with feature articles
3. Daily newsletters and bulletins for employees and management
4. High blood pressure bulletins and/or personal letters inserted in pay envelopes
5. Letters to employees' homes
6. Specially designed displays, which can be constructed inexpensively by the nurse and placed for maximum exposure
7. Mini high blood pressure presentations provided by the company's medical-nursing staff, perhaps in the cafeteria at convenient times
8. A free, convenient, and short slide session about high blood pressure
9. Local radio and community activity calendars

If applicable, union leadership can be requested to further promote the prescreening publicity. Their approval, input, and active visible assistance can be elicited initially and throughout the program to increase the potential for success.

Considerable emphasis may be placed on the voluntary and confidential aspects of the hypertension control program. It must be emphatically clear that no employee is forced to participate, that this is a free service of the health department, and not a requirement of the job. Strict confidentiality of all medical information obtained must be assured. Employees may not participate unless they feel secure that the information would not be used against them in terms of continued employment, promotion, or insurability. Union leadership can be instrumental in developing and approving the program and imparting this approval to employees.

Scheduled screening activities

Large scale company blood pressure screenings probably need to be done on an annual basis. Smaller programs can be conducted on an ongoing basis if blood pressure checks are not routine care, depending on the company's needs. In terms of the screening arrangements, scheduled appointments may be more convenient. Minimizing lost job time, production, and overtime costs by screening only a few people from any one area at a time is an excellent selling point to management. A "traveling blood pressure team" that screens employees at multiple locations within the industry is another viable alternative. If lost job time is a serious problem, blood pressure screening can be performed before or after work and during break and lunch times. Appointments may be scheduled directly or indirectly with the nurse or health office or through the supervisor.

Scheduling 10 to 20 people an hour is probably most efficient. Adequate counseling time for those with elevated blood pressure is crucial and must be considered in scheduling. The hours, departments, and sites can be adjusted to provide for adequate shift coverage. For example, a variety of hours, departments, and sites per 24-hour period for 1 week's duration may be adequate in a large company. Smaller companies require less. If an individual misses an appointment, it is necessary that he be contacted for rescheduling.

The blood pressure screening process was defined in Chapter 8. Variation of the procedures that the Milwaukee Blood Pressure Program utilizes may be necessary to meet an individual company's needs; however, the essential features remain the same.

In terms of physical facilities for screening, for one observer, two chairs, a table, standard sphygmomanometer, stethoscope, and a semiprivate location to protect confidentiality are required. An area free from noise and other extraneous distractions will enhance the accuracy of the blood pressure measurement.

Blood pressure screeners are trained and supervised by the professional nurse. Volunteers from the plant, community service organizations, American Heart Association, or other nursing services can be utilized. Frequent breaks or rest periods to prevent fatigue and reduce screener error are necessary.

Medical referral procedures

The blood pressure criteria for referral as described earlier may be utilized. Additionally, any screened individual with a diastolic level greater than 120 mm. Hg or with a 110 mm. Hg diastolic reading who is experiencing dizziness, headache, chest pains, shortness of breath, or any other symptoms of severe or malignant hypertension warrants immediate referral to medical care. This mechanism includes the options described previously or defined by the physician.

The individual with a normal blood pressure reading can be informed of his blood pressure reading as it compares to the criteria and be provided with an explanation of blood pressure and hypertension and the need for yearly blood pressure checks. Also a recheck card with the written date and latest blood pressure reading, hypertension pamphlets, and a brochure explaining the company's high blood pressure program can be distributed at the screening.

Second and third blood pressure screenings, on separate days within a 2-week period, can be performed at the company health department or other designated plant sites.

With a second elevated reading, a referral to the employee's physician for further evaluation is necessary. The company nurse can assist with the client's permission by calling the private physician to schedule the appointment to ensure follow through. If no personal physician is available, all efforts can be made to provide that individual with names of physicians accepting new patients. The local Medical Society will be helpful in this regard. The emphasis is the *need* for medical care and the *motivational* techniques that can be utilized to direct the client appropriately. If there is a treatment component to a particular company's· hypertension control program, the procedures defined for employee entry can be utilized.

Follow-up of employees with elevated blood pressure

Employee follow-up procedures are developed prior to initiating a screening program. Several approaches are utilized.

For example, the suspected hypertensive person can be given a form with the blood pressure reading information for the referring physician to complete. This form requests information regarding the individual's medical evaluation and therapy. The physician also is asked whether the company medical office can furnish hypertension education services and blood pressure monitoring between visits. This can be returned to the company nurse and documented on the individual's house records.

Or the aforementioned form can be sent directly to the physician. It can be requested to be returned to the company nurse for follow-up.

If the company nurse made the appointment with the private physician for the employee, that physician is contacted directly by the nurse periodically for follow-up. If the patient is noncompliant, collaborative efforts aggressively directed at motivating compliance may be initiated by the company nurse and private physician.

The Milwaukee Blood Pressure Program follow-up system consists of the following measures:

1. The private physician is telephoned with the client's approval to make an appointment. The client is present if possible.
2. A postcard is sent to the private physician with information on the blood pressure level and the dipstick urinalysis results. Just prior to the scheduled appointment, a follow-up card is sent to the physician requesting information about the patient on the last date seen, including blood pressure levels, drugs prescribed, complications present, and need for assistance with hypertension education. This can then be completed at the time of the visit or shortly thereafter.
3. If within a week after the appointment the information is not returned, the physician's office is telephoned and the information requested. Three months later and then annually this follow-up information is solicited. This type of patient monitoring system would facilitate the nurse's role in promoting patient compliance in an industrial setting.

A separate, confidential master index of all hypertensive patients with identifying information, blood pressure readings and dates, clinic visits, and educational summary is developed. If an employee is experiencing problems relating to the antihypertensive medication between visits, the nurse may consider contacting the private physician for drug adjustments and directions. Also the blood pressure recheck wallet card, which is issued to the patient with the first elevated blood pressure reading, is an extremely useful tool. This personal patient record is then brought to each physician or clinic visit and can be used by the industrial nurse to monitor the patient's progress and follow-up.

Hypertension education program

The hypertension education services that the industrial nurse can strategically provide may further enhance patient understanding, motivation, and hopefully compliance. As discussed in earlier chapters, in the therapeutic relationship, the nurse and medical department can effectively impart the genuine and personal interest and motivation necessary to support the hypertensive employee. Educational approaches such as the following may be undertaken:

1. Hypertension education series on an ongoing basis
2. Mini talks during scheduled breaks or lunchtime
3. Small group sessions
4. Panel discussions
5. Family high blood pressure classes or evening sessions
6. Posters and signs
7. Pamphlets and brochure distribution
8. Individual counseling initiated by the nurse
9. Audiovisual aides such as slides, tapes, and movies
10. Health fairs with high blood pressure as the central theme
11. Union-sponsored activities

A MODEL WORKSITE HYPERTENSION CONTROL PROGRAM

Alderman[1] has developed successful programs in New York City for treating hypertension at the worksite. Registered nurses and supervised paraprofessionals manage hypertensive patients within a protocol format. With this system, 81% of hypertensives treated were reported to have adequate blood pressure control. This approach to hypertension treatment appears to be appropriate and highly effective.

The Milwaukee Blood Pressure Program has developed and implemented a pilot university hypertension screening and treatment program collaboratively with the University of Wisconsin–Milwaukee Student Health Services. This innovative approach to hypertension control was generated out of increasing concern for the large number of late adolescent and young adults with undetected and untreated labile or essential hypertension. Since young adult men do not seek out medical care as often as women or the older population, this group is in particular jeopardy. Hypertension control services are brought to the young people rather than young people to the health care system.

The University of Wisconsin–Milwaukee is a large urban campus with approximately 30,000 students, faculty, and staff. Based on the worksite concept the Student Health Services is an ideal place, since the location is convenient, the hours are flexible for student needs, and the cost is minimal and appropriated from student fees and university funding. Also, this health care team addresses the unique needs and problems of the student population.

The essential components of the hypertension screening and treatment project are as follows:

1. Periodic screening of the students, faculty, and employees for hypertension
2. Physician referral, blood pressure monitoring, and renewal of antihypertensive prescriptions for well-controlled hypertensives in cooperation with practicing physicians
3. A campus hypertension treatment service for students who are unable to afford private physician care
4. Development of a hypertension and cardiovascular risk factor education program for the university community
5. Development of a system in patient tracking for long-term follow-up of hypertensive individuals being treated at the University of Wisconsin–Milwaukee
6. Acquisition of a data base for epidemiologic research in hypertension

Development of the program

Phase I. Phase I of the project, or the screening component, consisted of negotiating a collaborative relationship with the Student Health Services. The proposal was enthusiastically welcomed. The consideration and support received was the cornerstone for the success of the project. Also, the commitment of the student health center to quality health care for students was instrumental. Appropriate university administrative approval was obtained. Initially the Medical Society voiced concerns regarding the extent and purpose of the project. After discussion and clarification, the following guidelines were delineated:

1. Students with elevated blood pressure readings will be referred first to their private physicians.
2. Students who do not have a private physician, cannot afford, or do not desire private care at this time may elect to be treated at the student health center.
3. Students under private physician care will be provided free blood pressure monitoring and prescription renewal as the private physician requests.
4. University faculty and staff will not be provided long-term hypertension treatment. Considerable efforts are made to refer these individuals to private care. Blood pressure monitoring services and hypertension counseling may be provided.

Phase I also comprised the selection of campus screening sites and prescreening publicity and education. Campus sites were selected after carefully studying people-traffic patterns, convenience, accessibility, and hours of peak usage.

The suitability of the potential sites for blood pressure screening was determined by evaluating the noise levels, privacy, furniture arrangements, and fire department regulations. The student union, library, education, nursing, biological sciences, and business buildings were chosen. The student health center was designated as the primary screening operation site, with all second and third screens scheduled to return there.

The prescreening publicity and education component was initiated a month prior to the screening. The majority of the publicity was delivered during the week prior to and during the actual screening. Vehicles used to publicize the campaign included the following:

1. Posters and signs
2. Student handbills and pamphlets
3. Student, faculty, college and individual department, and general campus newspapers
4. Student organizations
5. Announcements by faculty and/or students during classes
6. Local community newspapers
7. Community and city radio news
8. Television coverage

Requests for volunteer support to assist with the mass screening were publicized. Volunteers from the following groups participated: campus student organizations, campus college of nursing and local nursing schools, American Heart Association, American Red Cross, city of Milwaukee, Medical College of Wisconsin, and others. A volunteer training manual and education series were utilized. The training sessions were conducted 2 weeks prior to the screening. Blood pressure measurement technique and the screening process were taught. Lectures, written materials, diagrams, films, audio cassettes, and several return demonstration sessions were utilized. Additionally, on site direction, reinforcement, and surveillance of volunteers ensured accuracy. Volunteers always participated under the supervision of the Milwaukee Blood Pressure Program staff and were not left unattended on site. All blood pressure elevations and any other problems were referred to the Milwaukee Blood Pressure Program staff. Many of these individuals offered their services for subsequent blood pressure screening projects.

The master scheduling, coordination, and placement of volunteers were successfully managed through the administrative office of the Milwaukee Blood Pressure Program. The program staff was scheduled for 3- to 6-hour periods with frequent breaks to prevent fatigue. Volunteers were scheduled similarly for 2-hour periods. Alternate plans were drawn to provide adequate site coverage for volunteer absences or failure to keep scheduled hours.

During the 2 weeks of mass campus screening, 5879 individuals were screened (Fig. 11). Cumulative data revealed that 83% of the population had normal blood pressure. Eight percent were considered to have labile hyperten-

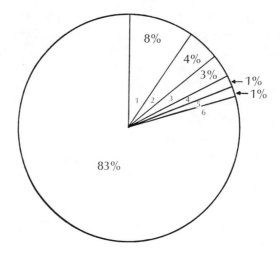

Fig. 11. Prevalence of hypertension among students at the University of Wisconsin at Milwaukee. BP ≥ 140/90 mm. Hg. N = 5879. *1,* Labile hypertension; *2,* newly detected hypertension; *3,* previously diagnosed but untreated hypertension; *4,* inadequate control; *5,* adequate control; *6,* normal blood pressure.

sion. These included individuals who previously were told by their physicians that they had high blood pressure but were found to have normal blood pressure on screening and those with elevated blood pressure readings on one screening but a normal reading on two subsequent screenings. Nine percent of the population were found to have sustained hypertension. At the time of screening, only 2% of the population said that they were receiving treatment. However, half the number had elevated blood pressure levels despite treatment. Four percent were found to be hypertensive without previous knowledge of the condition. Three percent were aware of their hypertension and were confirmed to have an elevated blood pressure but were not on therapy.

The statistical analysis of age, race, and sex categories did not reveal any significant difference.

One hundred and sixteen students with two elevated readings were referred to their private physicians for treatment. Eighty-seven students elected to be treated at the Student Health Services for the evaluation and management of hypertension.

Phase II. Phase II, or the treatment component, was initiated with a series of health center staff meetings to formulate clinic arrangements and educational services. Hypertension in-service sessions were also conducted. The director of the student health center designated which staff would be directly involved in the model clinic. The two registered nurses and one physician were selected to manage the clinic and were collaborated with closely.

The hypertension clinic is conducted one afternoon per week. At the second elevated screening, an appointment is made with the student health clinic, and an orientation pamphlet is issued. This summarizes the clinic operation for the student. The initial visits are scheduled at 15-minute intervals, which allows a nurse 30 minutes to obtain the history. Follow-up visits are scheduled at 10-minute intervals.

The clinic operates in the following manner. After clinic registration, the student is interviewed by the nurse. The history obtained also incorporates appropriate counseling. The physical parameters of height, weight, body frame, pulse, and blood pressure are measured by the nurse. The screening blood pressure readings and the results of the dipstick urinalysis are documented in the patient record. A physical examination is performed by the medical staff. Laboratory and other tests are ordered by the physician as indicated. Simple laboratory tests are processed at the student health center. All other laboratory and radiologic procedures are referred to a private community hospital in close proximity to the university.

The physician's evaluation of the student's condition and the plan of medical care with alternatives are discussed in detail with the patient. The therapy is prescribed utilizing the medication protocol described in Chapter 5. Initially the medications were dispensed to the student on a cost-free basis; however, budgetary restrictions necessitated modification of this practice. The commonly prescribed antihypertensives are dispensed at the health center at cost. Samples are distributed as available.

The student returns to the same nurse for an exit interview, education session, and appointment scheduling. Additional educational materials about hypertension specific to the college population in the written and audiovisual format are in the process of development and testing. Data generated from the initial evaluation are presented in Tables 5 to 8.

Follow-up visits consist of an entry and exit interview by the nurse and a physician examination. The physical parameters described earlier are again measured with the exception of height and body frame. Drug therapy and compliance are closely monitored, and therapy altered as necessary. Hypertension

Table 5. Initial blood pressure range (N = 65)

	Blood pressure (mm. Hg)	Number of patients	Percent
Normal blood pressure	≤140/90	15	23
Mild hypertension	140/90-154/104	37	56
Moderate hypertension	155/105-169/119	11	17
Severe hypertension	≥170/120	2	4

Table 6. Initial weight categories (N = 65)

	Number of patients	Percent
Normal	21	32
≤20% overweight	35	54
>20% overweight	9	14

Table 7. Diagnosis (N = 65)

	Number of patients	Percent
Normotensive	0	0
Labile hypertension	33	51
Essential hypertension	30	46
Secondary hypertension	2	3

Table 8. Follow-up data on students referred to practicing physicians for treatment of hypertension (N = 116)

	Number of patients	Percent
Drug therapy not initiated	44	39
Antihypertensive therapy initiated	47	41
Appointment failures	14	12
No physician response	11	9

counseling and risk factor modification are evaluated, repeated, and reinforced as necessary with the strategies discussed previously.

The outreach program for appointment reminders and failures is essentially the same as described in Chapter 8. The difference is a greater emphasis on confidentiality, especially if the student resides with his family or other roommates. Long-term tracking has been developed whereby the student's progress is followed after graduation and into employment. This consists of assisting the student to continue medical care by acquiring private physician care. That physician is then contacted periodically for information regarding the patient's progress. If the place of employment has a health department, the former student is encouraged to have his blood pressure monitored there. Additional long-term tracking services are being developed.

Collaboration with various university staff and departments such as psychology, athletic, and social work is essential to better address student needs. New avenues for research in various aspects of hypertension, such as studying the relaxation response for labile hypertensives in association with the psychology department and effects of alcohol consumption, have been initiated.

SUMMARY

High blood pressure screening and treatment at the worksite has proved to be a highly effective and readily adaptable approach to hypertension control. Advantages to both employer and employee are numerous. The industrial health department is in a strategic position to detect, monitor (possibly manage), and educate their respective hypertensive populations. The occupational nurse can catalyze the development of these types of services. The essential components of a hypertension control program in industry are as follows:

1. Prescreening publicity and education
2. Scheduled screening component
3. Referral for medical care and the follow-up of hypertensive employees
4. Hypertension education services
5. Treatment and monitoring of diagnosed hypertensives (optional)

Various approaches can be implemented for each component, depending on the industry's needs, resources, and commitment. A new tool to reach the hypertensive young adult population is hypertension screening and treatment in the campus setting. The worksite treatment concept promises dramatic opportunities for hypertension control and education.

SUGGESTED READINGS

1. Alderman, M. H.: Detection and treatment of hypertension at the work site. N. Engl. J. Med. **293**:65-68, 1975.
2. Charman, R. C.: Hypertension management program in an industrial community, J.A.M.A. **227**:288-291, 1974.
3. High blood pressure control in the work setting: issues, models, resources. In the Proceedings of the National Conference on High Blood Pressure, Oct. 14, 1976, West Point, Pa., 1977, Merck, Sharp & Dohme.
4. Hypertension at the work site: literature review and bibliography, reviewed by the National High Blood Pressure Education Program, National Institutes of Health, U.S. Department of Health, Education, and Welfare, March 1, 1976.
5. Hoover, W. A.: The future of occupational health programs, J. Occup. Med. **15**:483-485, 1973.
6. Schoenberger, J. A.: How industry can cut costs of employee heart attacks, Commerce, June, 1968.
7. Warshaw, L. J.: Insurance, occupational health and hypertension, Report of Proceedings of the National Conference on High Blood Pressure Education, DHEW Pub. No. (NIH) 73-486, pp. 91-94, Jan. 15, 1973.

Quality assurance—nursing outcomes for hypertension counseling

A quality assurance program evaluating a hypertension counseling program in terms of nursing outcomes is necessary. The program presented here is based on the educational services delivered by the professional nurses in our clinical settings.

The complete report of the Task Force on the Role of Nursing in High Blood Pressure Control (DHEW Pub. No. [NIH] 77-1241) became available in January 1978. This is an excellent resource and can be consulted as desired. Most of the goals, behavioral objectives (performance and cognitive skills), and attitude parameters are incorporated throughout the chapters. They may be adapted and applied to individual quality assurance programs.

NURSING OUTCOMES

I. During the detection process the nurse
1. Prepares and publicizes advance hypertension screening and education information
2. Develops hypertension educational materials appropriate to the needs of the community
3. Conveys the following information in the hypertension education program
   a. Defines blood pressure in systolic and diastolic terms
   b. Defines hypertension
   c. Describes the procedure for blood pressure measurement
   d. Identifies the prevalence of hypertension
   e. Explains the risks of hypertension in terms of family history, age, blood pressure levels, smoking, and weight
   f. Relates the silent and progressive nature of hypertensive disease
   g. Emphasizes the need for medical care
4. Employs motivational strategies to encourage blood pressure checks and medical referral where indicated
5. Tracks and performs follow-up activities on all referred suspected hypertensives
6. Coordinates and supervises the involvement of paraprofessionals and nonprofessionals in the hypertension detection and education process
7. Evaluates and revises periodically the hypertension detection procedures and educational program
II. During the treatment component of hypertension control the nurse
1. Orients the patient and family to the hypertension control services
2. Performs an assessment of the patient and his family's learning ability and readiness, psychosocial adaptation, and life-style

3. Constructs on a collaborative basis appropriate teaching goals, plans, and interventions based on the assessment data and patient and family needs
4. Implements teaching plans and strategies
5. Evaluates and revises teaching goals and interventions
6. Emphasizes that the cause of essential hypertension is not known
7. Describes the pathophysiologic mechanisms and natural course of hypertension
8. Describes complications of hypertension in terms of heart failure, stroke, and kidney disease
9. Delineates the daily range of fluctuations and trends in blood pressure
10. Identifies what factors affect blood pressure
11. Details therapeutic goals and plans
    a. Explains prescribed therapeutic regimens in detail
    b. Negotiates therapeutic plans when appropriate
    c. Negotiates expectations and time framework for goal accomplishments and evaluates and revises accordingly
    d. Promotes confidence in the efficacy of therapy
12. Explains and assesses the risk factors and their significance for that individual patient
    a. Encourages the positive steps that the patient and his family can take to modify their risks for cardiovascular disease and hypertension
    b. Negotiates with the patient and family to determine goals and individualized programs for risk factor modification and evaluates and revises accordingly
13. Explains the incidence, risk, and pathophysiologic effects of oral contraceptives
    a. As physician directed, suggests alternate forms of birth control and the frequency of blood pressure checks
    b. Monitors the blood pressure levels of pregnant women and refers accordingly
14. Details the relationship between exercise and cardiovascular disease
    a. Emphasizes the need for good physical condition and exercise
    b. Describes the physiologic and blood pressure changes during exercise
    c. Differentiates between isotonic and isometric exercises
    d. Ascertains patient current exercise activities, perceptions, and priorities
    e. Lists appropriate isotonic exercises and discourages isometric exercises
    f. Collaboratively plans an accelerated exercise or conditioning program according to the physician prescription, incorporating patient preferences
    g. Assists the patient to implement the exercise program and evaluates and revises exercise program accordingly
    h. Advises caution during exercise with certain antihypertensive medications
15. Explains the relationship of stress to hypertension
    a. Defines stress and identifies the various responses to stress
    b. Identifies and reinforces the appropriate methods that the patient and family utilize to manage stress
    c. Identifies and explains inappropriate or unhealthy methods that the patient and family employ to manage stress
    d. Collaborates and suggests more appropriate ways to manage stress
    e. Evaluates stress management at each clinic visit; initiates and monitors appropriate referrals to resources, professionals, or agencies

16. Provides counseling regarding the modification of smoking practices
    a. Assesses current smoking patterns at each clinic visit
    b. Quantitates the number of packages of cigarettes smoked daily and assigns patient consumption to the following defined risk categories
       (1) None or occasional cigarette smoker
           (a) Explains pathophysiologic effects of smoking
           (b) Defines smoking as a cardiovascular and pulmonary risk factor
           (c) Clarifies additional cardiovascular risks with presence of hypertension
           (d) Provides positive reinforcement for minimal or nonsmoking habits
       (2) Smokes less than one pack per day
           (a) Proceeds with the first three steps defined in the first category
           (b) Promotes self-evaluation on the part of the patient by attempting to explore the reasons for the smoking practices; ascertains patient priorities and desire to modify them
           (c) Jointly explores acceptable methods for decreasing smoking practices with the goal of eventual elimination
           (d) Employs appropriate motivational and educational strategies
           (e) Suggests antismoking group classes
           (f) Provides liberal positive reinforcement and support
           (g) Encourages family participation
           (h) Evaluates and revises strategies at each clinic visit
       (3) Smokes more than one pack per day
           (a) Proceeds with all steps defined in the first two categories
           (b) Provides stronger emphasis, guidance, and support to decrease or eliminate smoking habits
III. Counseling regarding the modification of dietary practices
    1. For salt (sodium)-intake modification the nurse
       a. Defines salt and its qualities
       b. Explains the relationship of salt and its effect on hypertension in terms of the following
          (1) Water retention
          (2) Effects on blood pressure
          (3) Usage with diuretics
       c. Assesses daily salt intake patterns
       d. Emphasizes the need for salt modification practices and collaboratively designs an individualized salt modification diet
       e. Lists foods to avoid and foods that are appropriate; advises the use of alternate herbs, spices, and salt substitutes
       f. Describes low-sodium cooking methods
       g. Describes the management of restaurant eating
       h. Explains how to determine sodium content in foods
       i. Provides printed and audiovisual material according to the patient's abilities
       j. Monitors salt intake at each clinic visit and documents the progress
       k. Clarifies, reinforces, and reviews counseling as necessary
    2. For potassium-intake modification, the nurse
       a. Defines potassium and its qualities and assesses dietary intake

    b. Explains the effect of diuretics on potassium levels in the body and their mechanism of action

    c. Collaborates and designs an individualized potassium-rich diet, and emphasizes the need for a potassium-rich diet

    d. Lists supplemental foods for daily consumption to augment potassium

    e. Provides printed and audiovisual materials according to the patient's ability

    f. Monitors potassium intake at each clinic visit and documents the progress

    g. Provides extensive counseling for the patient receiving supplemental potassium

    h. Monitors laboratory values and physical symptoms for potassium levels

    i. Alters the potassium-rich diet and medications based on the patient's clinical condition

3. For a low-fat diet the nurse
   a. Defines cholesterol and triglycerides and their effect on the circulatory system and blood pressure
   b. Defines atherosclerosis and its relationship to hypertension
   c. Describes the need for a low-fat diet
   d. Employs appropriate motivational strategies
   e. Differentiates between saturated and polyunsaturated fats
   f. Lists saturated and polyunsaturated fats as to their appropriateness
   g. Delineates guidelines for the low-fat diet
   h. Details the management of restaurant eating
   i. Explains low-fat cooking methods
   j. Discusses food planning, budgeting, buying, and labeling
   k. Jointly designs an individualized low-fat diet based on the nutritional assessment
   l. Provides printed and audiovisual materials according to the patient's ability
   m. Monitors the low-fat diet at each clinic visit and documents the progress
   n. Revises and alters the low-fat diet according to the patient's progress

4. Regarding weight control or loss the nurse
   a. Measures and documents the physical parameters of height, weight, and body frame
   b. Compares the measurements with the actuarial tables
   c. Informs the patient of weight status
   d. Explores and determines the need for weight loss with the patient sensitively
   e. Relates excess weight as a risk factor with hypertension
   f. Describes the physiologic effects of excess weight
   g. Employs motivational strategies to encourage the patient to participate in a weight loss program
   h. Respects the patient's decision regarding weight loss; if the patient elects not to lose weight at this time, other patient priorities are addressed and additional encouragement for weight loss is provided when appropriate
   i. Proceeds to initiate the following if the patient decides to engage in a weight loss program
      (1) Performs a 24-hour recall nutritional assessment as baseline data
      (2) Counsels regarding the basic four food groups (dairy products, meats,

fruits and vegetables, and breads and cereals), emphasizing low calorie, low-salt, and low-cholesterol food

(3) Discusses additional factors such as meal planning and scheduling, the rate of weight loss, the preparation and storage of food, and the management of restaurant eating and attempts to enlist family support and participation

(4) Utilizes individualized teaching interventions based on the patient's educational abilities and needs

(5) At each clinic visit, monitors basic four food groups daily intake, meal planning and scheduling, rate of weight loss or gain, preparation and storage of foods, family support and participation, salt-intake modification, and low-calorie and low-cholesterol foods; structured and supportive weight reduction groups are suggested if the patient would like to participate

5. For alcohol consumption modification the nurse
   a. Assesses current alcohol consumption at each clinic visit
   b. Quantitates alcohol consumption and assigns the patient to defined risk categories
   c. Explains the effects and consequences of alcohol consumption
   d. Defines additional cardiovascular risks with hypertension
   e. Jointly explores with the patient his needs and motivations for the alcohol intake
   f. Utilizes motivational strategies
   g. Assists patient to decrease alcohol consumption if desired by collaboratively outlining individualized methods
   h. Refers patient to appropriate community agencies
   i. Initiates and coordinates physician and resource follow-up

APPENDIX **B**

Hypertension patient education series

The hypertension education series presented here was developed for the newly diagnosed hypertensive patient initiated on treatment. The level of content is directed in a simple narrative fashion at the sixth grade level of comprehension for inner-city clientele. All artwork and designs have been deleted to conserve space and to enhance the adaptability of this tool. This information can be utilized in booklet, flip chart, audio cassette, poster, or other formats as we have done in our clinical settings. Much of the information is included in Chapter 6. The educational theory and nursing process basis are also discussed in Chapter 6.

THE PATIENT PAMPHLET

1. **Why is everyone talking about high blood pressure?**
   Because 50 million Americans may have hypertension, commonly called "high blood pressure." More than a fourth of these people don't know they have it and less than half are being treated. Over 30 billion dollars is spent every year on the consequences of high blood pressure like heart failure, stroke, or kidney disease.

2. **What is blood pressure?**
   Blood pressure is the force of blood pressing against the blood vessel wall. The heart is the muscle pumping the blood through the body. When the heart is squeezing or pumping, there is greater pressure or force pushing the blood through the blood vessel. This is called the "systolic blood pressure," or the top number in the blood pressure reading. When the heart is resting between beats, there is less pressure in the blood vessel. This is called the "diastolic blood pressure," or the bottom number in the blood pressure reading. In some people the blood pressure goes up and stays up most of the time. This is called "high blood pressure," or "hypertension." Hypertension, then, is continuous high blood pressure. Most individuals who have high blood pressure have the *essential* type. The cause of essential hypertension is not known at this time.

3. **How do I know if I have high blood pressure?**
   By getting your blood pressure checked every year. This is important because hypertension is a silent disease. There is no characteristic or any certain set of symptoms. Headache, dizziness, shortness of breath, flushing, or tingling may be from high blood pressure. They may also be caused by other health problems, so a doctor's evaluation is necessary. These symptoms may be warning signs before a major problem occurs. Also, being a progressive disease, the damage occurs slowly and continuously over a period of time, especially if not treated; so long-term care is abso-

191

lutely necessary. This means it is very important to get under and stay with a doctor's care.

4. Who gets high blood pressure?

Anyone at any age can have high blood pressure. Doctors have found that more men have hypertension than women and more blacks than whites. Even slightly higher blood pressure readings in young persons can mean serious problems later. Also, being overweight, eating too much salt, and having stressful problems can cause the high blood pressure to appear sooner and be higher.

5. What is a normal blood pressure reading?

Your doctor or nurse can tell you what your "normal" blood pressure is, so be sure to ask. Remember—the higher the blood pressure level the more serious the risk of early death and complications such as heart failure, stroke, and kidney disease.

6. What if someone in my family has high blood pressure?

If someone in your family has high blood pressure, heart problems, stroke, or kidney disease, that may mean a greater risk for you having hypertension. So getting your blood pressure checked every year is a family affair.

7. How can high blood pressure cause the following conditions?

Heart failure. High blood pressure can cause heart failure by straining the heart. With high blood pressure, the heart must pump against such high pressure that it becomes overworked. The heart muscles become thicker and larger to pump harder and faster. Eventually the heart becomes so thick and weak that it cannot pump enough blood. Worse yet, blood vessels surrounding the heart may have atherosclerosis (clumps of fat that stick to the blood vessel wall), which further damages the heart and causes heart failure. The signs of heart failure may be swollen or puffy ankles, weight gain, and shortness of breath.

Stroke. High blood pressure can also damage your brain. This happens by the high blood pressure of blood causing the blood vessels in the brain to lose their ability to stretch, and they get weak. The blood vessels in the brain are fragile and sensitive. When the blood vessels get weak enough from the atherosclerosis and high blood pressure, they break and bleed into the brain. This is a stroke and can cause paralysis, which means no feeling or movement of arms and legs. The signs of stroke may be headache, dizziness, and numbness or weakness in arms or legs.

Kidney disease. The kidneys filter out wastes from the blood. High blood pressure damages these tiny blood vessels, and the kidneys can no longer filter out the wastes in your body. This is very serious. Some signs may be blood in the urine or a change in your usual urine or water habits.

Eye changes. High blood pressure weakens and can damage the blood vessels behind the eye. This is partly why the doctor checks your eyes routinely. Some signs of eye changes may be blurring or seeing spots.

The important point to remember is that hypertension is serious and you need to get under and stay with medical care. Taking your medicine as ordered and following your doctor or nurse's advice will control your blood pressure and prevent or slow down many of these problems.

8. How does the doctor treat high blood pressure?

Each person with high blood pressure is different, so treatment depends on your doctor's evaluation. The important points to remember are

a. Continue to see your doctor or nurse regularly.

b. Take your medications as ordered.

c. Follow your doctor or nurse's advice about the changes in your life-style.

9. **What about smoking and high blood pressure?**

Don't smoke, if possible. Smoking makes the heart beat faster, raises your blood pressure, upsets the flow of blood and air in the lungs, and damages the lining of the lungs. The constant strain that smoking, high-fat diet, and high blood pressure place on the heart adds up and is deadly. Following are some ways to begin "kicking the habit":

a. Choose a cigarette with less tar and nicotine.

b. Smoke only the first half of the cigarette.

c. Reduce the number of times a puff is taken on the cigarette.

d. Reduce the depth of inhalation.

e. Smoke fewer cigarettes a day.

f. Exercise more.

g. Pursue new hobbies and interests.

h. Find a safe substitute for handling cigarettes like a lucky coin, pen, or pencil.

Sometimes people who are trying to quit smoking begin to gain weight. Keeping low-calorie foods and beverages within easy reach helps instead of a cigarette.

10. **What about alcohol and high blood pressure?**

Drinking alcohol is a risk with high blood pressure. Although the first drink may lower the blood pressure a little, it will rise with more alcohol. Heavy weekend drinking can be a real problem. Large amounts of alcohol, especially over a short period of time, in an individual with high blood pressure places a tremendous strain on the heart and circulation. In addition, alcohol and high blood pressure medications can be a dangerous combination. So take your medicine daily and limit your drinking. Try the following suggestions:

a. Drink low-calorie beer.

b. Limit the number and kind of drinks. In other words, have fewer drinks and avoid strong liquors.

c. Buy smaller amounts.

d. Drink other beverages like coffee, soda, milk, tea, or fruit juice.

11. **Can exercise affect high blood pressure?**

Everyone needs some type of exercise daily. If you have hypertension or other health problems, ask your doctor's advice before starting an exercise program. A slowly advanced or step-by-step approach to exercising is usually advised. An example may be to start walking two blocks a day and slowly add on more blocks and speed until you are jogging a mile a day, but this depends on your doctor's orders. Generally speaking, exercises like running, walking, swimming, or bicycling lower your blood pressure and are very good. These are called "isotonic" types of exercise. But exercises like pressing weights or lifting heavy objects can cause a very high and fast blood pressure change. These are called "isometric" types of exercises and can be avoided. Also, certain high blood pressure medicines, which are discussed later in this pamphlet, can change your body's response to exercise or fast position changes. You may feel weak, faint, or dizzy. When this happens, stop the exercise and slow down your fast movements and be sure to tell your doctor or nurse and follow their advice.

12. **What about stress and high blood pressure?**

Stress is any situation that creates an uncomfortable feeling, tension, or strain in the person. Each person sees and handles stress differently. Stressful situations usually mean a change or adjustment. Stressful situations may be positive or negative (good or bad) like marriage, birth of a child, new job, or death of a loved one. In these situations or even when hungry or rushing to work, the blood pressure rises and the heart beats faster for a short time, but your blood pressure will rise even higher. Your brain, heart, and kidneys need to be protected against that. The following advice may help you handle the stress differently:

a. Look at the problem or stressful situation. Recognize your limits and that you are human.

b. What are your responses to the stress? Are they in your best personal and health interests?

c. Adapt to the stressful problem by thinking about and acting on alternatives or solutions.

d. Learn to relax.

13. **Why do my blood pressure numbers change? Sometimes it is 180/100 and other times it is 160/92.**

Everyone's blood pressure changes many times a day. For example, when you're sleeping, your blood pressure is lower. When you're awake, your blood pressure rises steadily throughout the day until early evening when it begins to lower. So expect some changes with your blood pressure readings. You can ask the doctor or nurse what these changes may be.

14. **What are some changes I can make in my diet to help control my high blood pressure?**

Diet changes are part of your total treatment plan to control your high blood pressure. Basically, you need to cut down on your salt and salty, fatty, or high cholesterol foods, and keep your weight under control. You may also need to lose weight. If you are taking diuretic medicine, you will need to eat more potassium-rich foods.

Let's start with the basic good diet that everyone needs daily:

a. Two or more servings of milk or dairy products every day

b. Two or more servings of meat or substitutes every day

c. Four or more servings of fruits and vegetables every day

d. Four or more servings of bread or cereals every day

Now let's talk about cutting down on salt and salty foods in your diet. Salt is a natural chemical called "sodium chloride," which is found in the human body, foods, and the oceans. Salt is best known as a spice; however, the sodium part of salt acts differently in the human body. There it holds water inside the body. The kidneys are the filters of the body and pass a certain amount of sodium and water out of the body in the urine every day. When more salt is eaten than the body needs, more water is held inside the body. With hypertension, the kidneys don't pass the salt and water out of the urine fast enough, and the blood pressure rises.

The diuretic or water pill that the doctor has prescribed to control your high blood pressure works with the kidneys to pass more salt and water out of the body in the urine. This is one way to keep the high blood pressure controlled. The diuretics work best with the kidneys if less salt is eaten with and in your foods. The easiest way to cut down on your salt is not to use salt during your cooking or at the table and to avoid salty foods.

Avoid these high-salt foods:

Meat group: Sausage, weiners, ham, bacon, corned beef, luncheon meats or cold cuts, saltpork, smoked fish, herring, sardines, canned meats, and TV dinners

Dairy group: Cheese or processed cheese and buttermilk

Fruit and vegetable group: Olives, pickles, sauerkraut, and canned vegetables

Snack foods: Potato chips, porkrinds, salted nuts, and salted popcorn

Seasonings: Salt, garlic or onion salt, boullion, soy sauce, and canned soups

Eat these low-salt foods as desired:

Meat and fish group: Poultry, fresh or frozen fish, veal, lamb, pork, and lean beef

Dairy group: Low-fat milk, low-fat cottage cheese, and ice milk

Fruit and vegetable group: Any fresh or frozen foods in this group

Bread and cereal group: Most commercial or baked breads or cereals

Snack foods: Sherbet, fruit ice, gelatin, and fruit drinks

Seasonings: Garlic, onion, bayleaf, pepper, dill, nutmeg, rosemary, green pepper, honey, lemon juice, etc.

Now you can begin to enjoy the "real" taste of foods, not just the condiments. One tip on preparing foods for a low-salt diet is use more fresh or frozen foods and avoid canned foods, which are high in salt. Also leftover cooking liquids can be used with soups or stews. An important shopping tip is to read the labels of foods and to look for the salt or sodium content. If the word "sodium" or "salt" is in the first four to five ingredients, avoid that food.

A tip for restaurant eating with a low-salt diet is to eat foods that are boiled, baked, broiled, or roasted without salted gravies or juices. Avoid soups and salted or cheese dressings. You can carry your own salt substitute or a special dressing.

15. What about a potassium-rich diet?

Potassium is a vital mineral in the body that is chemically a partner to salt. The diuretic medication prescribed passes more salt and water out of the body to control high blood pressure, but the potassium is washed out with the salt. So more high potassium foods need to be taken in the diet to put back the lost potassium. Most fresh fruits and vegetables are high in potassium and can be eaten three or four times a day. Foods such as bananas, oranges, and squash are especially helpful. Fruit juices are other important sources. A good suggestion is to have one or two fruits with the diuretic every morning.

16. What about a low-fat diet?

Generally, all animal fats are *saturated*. This includes milk, cream, cheese, butter, beef, and chicken fat. In addition, solid vegetable fat such as shortening and coconut oils is saturated. These saturated fats can raise blood cholesterol and fat, causing hardening of the arteries. This means that the arteries become stiffer and less movable. Also, plaques or clumps of fat stick to the wall of the blood vessel, making the inside rougher and smaller. This is called "atherosclerosis." Atherosclerosis makes it more difficult for the blood with nutrients and oxygen to pass and also raises the blood pressure. This is a risk with high blood pressure. Foods with saturated fats and cholesterol need to be avoided. Your body produces its own cholesterol, so lots of extra cholesterol in the diet is not needed.

Low-saturated fats or polyunsaturated fats generally include vegetable fats. These polyunsaturated fats lower blood cholesterol and are strongly advised. Some guidelines for low saturated fat diets include the following:

a. Use margarines or vegetable oils instead of butter.
b. Avoid gravies, creams, and cheese sauces.
c. Have eggs three to four times a week. (This varies with your doctor's orders.)
d. Drink skim milk and skim milk products.
e. Trim or skim fats from baked, broiled, or boiled meats or poultry. Avoid fried foods.
f. Enjoy fish, poultry, and veal more often. Beef, ham, and pork can be limited.

When buying foods it is important to read the labels for fat content and to buy foods that are made from polyunsaturated or vegetable fats. Also, buy leaner cuts of meat. Following are tips for low-fat cooking:

a. Trim off as much fat as possible.
b. Broil, roast, or bake the meat, using a wire rack so that the fat can drip off.
c. Boil or simmer, but immediately remove the meat from the cooking liquid.
d. Do not fry or deep-fat fry. You may sauté in a shallow Teflon-coated pan. For soups and gravies, chilling causes the fat to harden, which can be skimmed off.
e. Cut off all poultry skin.

17. What about weight and high blood pressure?

Being overweight is an added risk with high blood pressure. There are definitely more complications like heart failure, stroke, or diabetes in persons with high blood pressure who are overweight. It is very important to keep your weight under control and to lose weight if the doctor advises so. The two most important ways to lose weight are (a) begin new eating habits and (b) learn control. *Beginning new eating habits* means eating three balanced meals a day from the meat, dairy, bread, and fruit and vegetable groups, no snacking between meals except for acceptable low-calorie foods, and no meals 4 hours prior to evening sleep. *Learning control* means learning to limit the size and number of servings. Your rate of weight loss may be about 1 pound per week. Have low-calorie food around like fruits and vegetables, artificial sweeteners, coffee, tea, and sugarless candy.

18. What else should I know about high blood pressure treatment?

The goal of your therapy is to control your high blood pressure and prevent or slow down complications like heart failure, stroke, or kidney disease. The doctor will tell you what your controlled blood pressure should be. Once your blood pressure is controlled, do not stop taking the blood pressure medicine, thinking you are "cured." Therapy for high blood pressure is lifelong. At the present time, there is no "cure" for hypertension, but we can control high blood pressure. So you must keep taking medicines even if you feel well. Remember, taking medicine is a lot cheaper and less painful than heart failure or stroke.

Some people worry about being dependent on medicine or feel ashamed that they have a health problem. Thirty million other Americans have high blood pressure and that is no sign of weakness or inferiority. Certainly, not getting treatment is wrong.

Make very sure you understand the doctor or nurse's orders for taking the medicine. You need to know:

a. The name and type of drug and why you are taking it
b. The time of day and how many pills to take
c. Some side effects or temporary changes and what to do about them

So ask, because only your doctor or nurse can give you the exact information about your medicines.

Getting into a routine schedule like taking the pills on awakening from sleep, when brushing your teeth, or with breakfast helps. If you happen to miss a dose or two, that's okay, you're human. Just don't take the doses you missed as extra to make up for lost ones. Get back on your regular medication schedule.

19. Can you tell me more about high blood pressure medications?
Most cases of high blood pressure can be controlled with medication. It is absolutely necessary that you take the medication as ordered by your doctor or nurse every day. Since every patient with hypertension is different, the kind and dose of medicine prescribed for you is different. Because your body acts in a unique way with each drug, they may be changed or switched until your blood pressure is controlled. When you first start taking new medicines or new doses, you may feel some changes. These changes usually last for a short time or sometimes longer as your blood pressure and body adjust to the medicines. Be sure to tell the doctor or nurse about these changes so that they will know how the medicines are working. Never stop taking your prescribed medicines without your doctor or nurse's advice.

All patients are asked to bring to the clinic their pills and any other medicines that they have taken since the last appointment. This is because the doctor and nurse want to make sure you are taking the right medication the right way. Also, sometimes between visits patients get ill or for other reasons take other medicines. It is very important *not* to take other medicines without telling your doctor or nurse because they may interfere, block, or make you sick with the high blood pressure medicines. Generally, there are two kinds of high blood pressure medicine: diuretics and antihypertensives.

20. What are diuretics?
Diuretics are "water pills." Almost all patients with high blood pressure take diuretic medicine, which works with your kidneys to pass more salt and water out of the blood into the urine. This lowers blood pressure and is one way to keep the blood pressure controlled. Diuretics work best with the kidneys if you eat less salt and salty type foods.

You may be told to take the pills once or a couple of times a day. It is easier to take the diuretics in a routine, like in the morning with fruit juice at breakfast; or keep the pills with your toothbrush so you automatically take them when you brush your teeth. For the next few weeks you will pass more water or urinate more often. It is probably best not to take the diuretics close to sleep time. You may be awakened from sleep to go to the bathroom.

After you have been taking the diuretics for a while, you will not be passing as much urine as when you first started taking the pills. This is normal. The diuretics are still controlling your blood pressure and your body has adjusted to the medicine.

Sometimes patients feel some temporary changes or have mild side effects from the diuretic medicines. Expected temporary changes may be dry mouth or passing more urine. These are *not* serious, and most of them will disappear in time as your body and blood pressure adjust to the water pills. Side effects are changes caused by the diuretics that are not expected or normal. These may be drowsiness, muscle weakness, cramps, joint pains, or extreme thirst or hunger with weight loss. It is very important to call the clinic nurse or doctor should problems or questions occur and not to stop taking the medicine. Some common diuretics that may be prescribed are Esidrix, Hydrodiuril, or Hygroton.

21. Why do I need a potassium-rich diet or potassium medicine with the diuretic water pills?

Remember, diuretics pass more salt and water out of the body to control high blood pressure, but potassium, which is a mineral partner of salt, is washed out too. So all patients taking diuretics need foods that are rich in potassium like orange juice and bananas. Generally, most fresh fruits and vegetables are potassium rich and need to be eaten two to four times a day. For some patients, potassium medicine may be prescribed. This can be taken with or in fruit juice at the same time you take the water pills. If you feel an upset stomach, take more water with the potassium medicine and take the medicine with meals. If the upset stomach continues, be sure to tell the doctor or nurse. Sometimes, instead of prescribing potassium medicine, other diuretic medicines that stop the potassium from being washed out of your urine like Dyazide or Aldactazide may be used.

22. What are the other types of high blood pressure medicines?

With high blood pressure, several types of medicines may need to be taken every day. This team of medicines works well to control your hypertension. Besides diuretics, other members of the team of medicines that may be prescribed are nerve blockers and vasodilators. *Nerve blockers* work with the nerves surrounding your blood vessels. They are called "nerve blockers" because they block certain nerve messages and chemical changes so your blood vessels will open more. This lowers your blood pressure and keeps it controlled. These drugs are Aldomet, Aldoril, and others. *Vasodilators* such as hydralazine relax and open up your blood vessels, causing the blood pressure to go down.

You will probably take a combination of these medicines a couple of times a day with diuretics. Together this team of medicines will control your high blood pressure.

23. Will I feel some changes with these medicines?

When you first start taking the vasodilators or nerve blockers, you may feel somewhat dizzy, weak, or faint when standing or making fast body movements as in exercise. This is common and an expected temporary adjustment and will lessen after awhile; but with hot weather, with exercise, or after drinking alcohol you are especially prone to this. To prevent the dizziness, faintness, and/or weakness:

a. Slow down your body movements; for example, when you arise from bed in the morning first sit up at the side of the bed for a few moments. When you feel comfortable, begin to stand slowly.

b. Wear support stockings, which can be put on before getting up from bed in the morning.

c. Slow down your fast body movements or exercises. Your body will tell you how fast to move by beginning to feel weak or faint.

d. Sleep with the head of your bed raised about 6 inches with pillows or blocks.

When you feel weak, faint, or dizzy:

a. Sit or lie down and rest for awhile until the faintness passes.

b. Slowly begin moving again.

c. Be sure to tell your doctor or nurse.

d. Be patient with yourself.

When you begin taking vasodilators or nerve blockers, you may feel a bit tired or sleepy for awhile. If you have the kind of job in which you operate heavy machinery or drive a lot, it is important to know about the possible dizziness, sleepiness, or faintness to avoid accidents. *Use caution.* Changing the times for the medicine doses from the day to the evening hours after work and before sleep may be helpful. If these temporary changes do not disappear after a few weeks or are not tolerable for you, please call the clinic.

Some patients may have dry mouth, upset stomach, diarrhea, or constipation. Taking the medicine with meals and a lot of fluids helps to avoid these. These are side effects that the clinic doctor or nurse want to know about.

If you have a stuffy nose more often than usual, again be sure to tell your doctor or nurse. It is important to use caution with over-the-counter drugs for the stuffy nose, since these can raise your blood pressure.

If you notice that you are feeling "down," moody, more or less hungry, and are having problems sleeping, again be sure to tell the doctor or nurse. The drug will probably need to be changed.

At first, some men may feel changes when having sex. This may be in different ways, like the penis not getting as hard as usual or not being able to keep the hardness as long as before or the semen coming out differently. None of these changes are harmful or permanent and are usually lessened in time if you relax. You may want to talk this problem over with your sex partner. This can be very helpful. Be patient with yourself and tell your doctor or nurse about these problems.

So the important points to remember about the medications are:

a. Take the medication every day.

b. Realize that there may be some temporary changes and/or side effects as your blood pressure and body adjust.

c. Do not stop taking the medication without your doctor or nurse's advice.

d. Tell the doctor or nurse about any problems that you are having with the medicine.

e. Live your new life-style and enjoy it.

24. **What about birth control pills and high blood pressure?**

Women who take birth control pills double their chances for having high blood pressure. The exact reason is not known yet, but doctors do know that the hormones in the pills can cause the body to hold in more salt and water, which could raise the blood pressure. Be sure to tell your doctor if you or someone in your family has high blood pressure, heart or kidney problems, stroke, or diabetes. This may mean your chances for having hypertension are greater and perhaps another type of birth control is better for you, depending on your doctor's evaluation.

25. **If I am taking birth control pills or hormones for change of life, how will I know if I have high blood pressure?**

By seeing your doctor regularly and having your blood pressure checked every 3 months or as advised.

26. **What if I develop high blood pressure while on birth control pills or change-of-life hormones?**

    Your doctor will decide what is best for you. The doctor may stop the pills and prescribe different birth control methods or keep the pills and perhaps prescribe other medicines. In that case your blood pressure will be checked more often.

27. **Can I have high blood pressure if I am pregnant?**

    Yes, pregnant women can develop high blood pressure. This condition is also called "preeclampsia," or "toxemia." The exact cause is not known, but doctors do know that if you had high blood pressure before you were pregnant, your chances for developing high blood pressure complications during pregnancy is higher. You will need to visit the doctor more often and follow his advice closely.

28. **Are there some danger signs during pregnancy that can alert me to see my doctor?**

    Yes, contact your doctor if you have:
    - Headaches
    - Vision problems
    - Swelling of ankles, feet, hands, or puffy eyelids
    - More of a weight gain than prescribed

PATIENT EDUCATION AND RESPONSIBILITY EVALUATION

The following forms will be helpful to the nurse in evaluating the patient and significant others' understanding of hypertension education and their progress relating to incorporating life-style changes appropriate for self-care. Furthermore, the specific behavior objectives, consisting of performance and cognitive skills, and the attitude changes on the patient's part need to be individualized and prioritized. These can be delineated when appropriate and revised accordingly.

General hypertension information

Negotiated goals and priorities	P and SO* description	Dates		Dates		Negotiated nursing responsibility, motivational strategies, teaching interventions† (type, date, evaluation and signature)
		Negotiated patient responsibility	Today's results	Negotiated patient responsibility	Today's results	
	1. Defines blood pressure					
	2. Describes hypertension					

	3. Approximates rate of high blood pressure in United States (if applicable)
	  50 million Americans have high blood pressure
	  More men have hypertension than women
	  More blacks have hypertension than whites
	  Family history of high blood pressure, heart and kidney problems, or diabetes means more risk for high blood pressure
	  The higher the blood pressure reading, the more serious the risk of early death and complications like heart attack, stroke, or kidney disease
	  Silent disease without a "set" of symptoms					

*P = Patient; SO = significant others.

†Teaching interventions: 1 = individual counseling; 2 = written materials; 3 = audiovisual presentations; 4 = group sessions.

Continued.

General hypertension information—cont'd

Negotiated goals and priorities	P and SO* description	Dates		Dates		Negotiated nursing responsibility, motivational strategies, teaching interventions† (type, date, evaluation and signature)
		Negotiated patient responsibility	Today's results	Negotiated patient responsibility	Today's results	
	Physician's care is absolutely necessary, since hypertension is lifelong, causing continuous damage if not treated					
	4. Vocalizes that the cause of high blood pressure is not known, but most people have essential hypertension					
	5. Defines a risk factor as a condition that makes a person more prone to develop hypertension and have more severe high blood pressure					
	6. Relates that being overweight, eating too much salt, and having more stress problems causes the hypertension to appear sooner and more severely					
	7. Vocalizes that birth control pills may cause the blood pressure to rise (as applicable)					
	8. States that exercise like walking, swimming, running, and rhythm calisthenics are good for general					

body conditioning and high blood pressure					
9. Describes the need for good physical condition to keep the heart and body in shape					
10. Lists exercises such as weight lifting and pushing heavy objects as not the most beneficial types of physical activity with high blood pressure					
11. If on sympathetic inhibitor therapy, states that drugs which lower blood pressure (insert the name of the patient's drug) can cause dizziness and fainting with exercise and fast position changes					
12. Describes stress					
13. Vocalizes that stress may cause the blood pressure to rise					
14. Lists ways people can act under stress a. Ignore the situation and not feel the strain b. Divert their attention to another activity c. Face and accept the situation					

Continued.

General hypertension information—cont'd

Negotiated goals and priorities	P and SO* description	Dates		Dates		Negotiated nursing responsibility, motivational strategies, teaching interventions† (type, date, evaluation, and signature)
		Negotiated patient responsibility	Today's results	Negotiated patient responsibility	Today's results	
	d. Do nothing, but feel the strain					
	e. Seek help					
	15. States better ways to handle stress					
	a. See what the stress is or will be					
	b. Why is it stressful?					
	c. How would I or am I responding to the stress? Are these responses in my best personal and health interests?					
	d. Look at alternatives to handle and/or accept the situation					
	16. Explains that relaxation techniques may help lower blood pressure (only if applicable)					
	17. States the two major patient responsibilities of high blood pressure therapy:					
	a. To take medication every day					
	b. To continue with physician's care					
	18. Other					

Medication

Negotiated goals and priorities	P and SO* description	Dates			Dates			Negotiated nursing re-sponsibility, motiva-tional strategies, teach-ing interventions† (type, date, evaluation and signature)
		Negotiated patient re-sponsibility	Today's results		Negotiated patient re-sponsibility	Today's results		
	1. States the necessity of taking the medicine							
	2. Explains that the physician or nurse may change the medication as the blood pressure is controlled and body adjusts							
	3. Verbalizes that with new medication or new doses he may feel some temporary changes and/or side effects							
	4. Explains that he can call the physician or nurse about these changes and not to stop taking the medicine without the physician or nurse's advice							
	5. Defines the overall goal of high blood pressure therapy							
	6. Verbalizes that high blood pressure therapy does not "cure" but can control hy-pertension; therapy is life-long							

*P = Patient; SO = significant others.
†Teaching interventions: 1 = individual counseling; 2 = written material; 3 = audiovisual presentations; 4 = group sessions.

Continued.

Medication—cont'd

Negotiated goals and priorities	P and SO* description	Dates		Dates		Negotiated nursing responsibility, motivational strategies, teaching interventions† (type, date, evaluation and signature)
		Negotiated patient responsibility	Today's results	Negotiated patient responsibility	Today's results	
	7. Describes the importance of a routine medication schedule					
	8. Defines diuretics					
	9. Explains how they act to lower blood pressure					
	10. States need for low-salt diet with diuretics					
	11. Explains how he takes his pills					
	12. Briefly describes some temporary changes and side effects from diuretics					
	13. Explains what he would do if the changes or side effects occurred					
	14. Explains the need for a potassium-rich diet with diuretic medicine					
	15. Explains how he takes the potassium medicine (if applicable)					
	16. Describes the need to use a team of high blood pressure medicines					
	17. Explains how the following medications lower blood					

pressure (as applicable): vasodilators and nerve blockers		
18. Explains temporary changes as expected, mild and short-term; differentiates these from side effects and describes their management		
19. Describes what he would do if any of the following side effects occurred a. Upset stomach, diarrhea, or constipation b. Stuffy nose (frequent) c. Feeling down, moody, more or less hungry, or having sleeping problems d. Sexual problems		
20. Summarizes important points to remember about taking high blood pressure medicine a. Take as ordered by your doctor or nurse b. Realize there may be some temporary changes and/or side effects as your body adjusts c. Do not stop taking the medication without the physician or nurse's advice d. Tell the physician or nurse about any problems with the medication		

Low-sodium diet

Negotiated goals and priorities	P and SO* description	Dates		Dates		Negotiated nursing responsibility, motivational strategies, teaching interventions† (type, date, evaluation, and signature)
		Negotiated patient responsibility	Today's results	Negotiated patient responsibility	Today's results	
	1. Salt intake					
	a. Avoids extremely salty foods, and adds no salt during cooking or at the table					
	b. Adds some salt during cooking but not at the table					
	c. Salts foods during cooking and at table					
	2. Defines salt and its functions in the body					
	3. Explains how salt affects his blood pressure					
	4. Describes what high-salt intake can do with diuretic medication					
	5. Lists high-salt foods not to					

be eaten in each of the following: meat and fish group, dairy group, fruit and vegetable group, and bread and cereal group			
6. Lists low-salt foods			
7. Vocalizes his low-salt diet menus			
8. Explains low-salt cooking methods and his progress			
9. Describes how to manage restaurant eating with low-salt diet and his progress			
10. Describes how to look for sodium (salt) content by reading food labels and his progress			
11. What are the patient's perceptions and priorities relative to his salt consumption, needs, and desires?			
12. Other			

*P = Patient; SO = significant others.

†Teaching interventions: 1 = individual counseling; 2 = written materials; 3 = audiovisual presentations; 4 = group sessions.

High-potassium diet

Negotiated goals and priorities	P and SO* description	Dates			Dates			Negotiated nursing responsibility, motivational strategies, teaching interventions† (type, date, evaluation, and signature)
		Negotiated patient responsibility	Today's results		Negotiated patient responsibility	Today's results		
	1. Potassium intake: delineates number of potassium rich food servings per day							
	2. Describes how diuretic medications lower blood pressure							
	3. Explains the need for diuretic medication							
	4. Defines potassium and how diuretics lower blood potassium							
	5. Lists high-potassium foods to be eaten							
	6. Vocalizes his high-potassium food menu							
	7. What are the patient's perceptions relative to his potassium intake, needs, and desires?							
	8. Other							

*P = Patient; SO = significant others.

†Teaching interventions: 1 = individual counseling; 2 = written materials; 3 = audiovisual presentations; 4 = group sessions.

Low–saturated fat diet

Negotiated goals and priorities	P and SO* description	Dates		Dates		Negotiated nursing responsibility, motivational strategies, teaching interventions† (type, date, evaluation, and signature)
		Negotiated patient responsibility	Today's results	Negotiated patient responsibility	Today's results	
	1. Differentiates between saturated and polyunsaturated fats					
	2. Lists saturated fats					
	3. Lists polyunsaturated fats					
	4. Defines risks of high–saturated fat diet with high blood pressure					
	5. Describes atherosclerosis and risks with high blood pressure					
	6. States what cholesterol and triglycerides are and simply how the body acquires them					
	7. Explains ways to lessen blood cholesterol and triglycerides					
	8. States guidelines for low–saturated fat diet					
	9. Vocalizes his low–saturated fat menus					
	10. Describes how to read labels for fat content					
	11. Explains low-fat cooking methods					

*P = Patient; SO = significant others.

†Teaching interventions: 1 = individualized counseling; 2 = written materials; 3 = audiovisual presentations; 4 = group sessions.

Continued.

Low–saturated fat diet—cont'd

Negotiated goals and priorities	P and SO* description	Dates		Dates		Negotiated nursing responsibility, motivational strategies, teaching interventions† (type, date, evaluation and signature)
		Negotiated patient responsibility	Today's results	Negotiated patient responsibility	Today's results	
	12. Lists food buying and budgeting hints for low-fat diet					
	13. What are the patient perceptions, priorities, needs, and desires relative to his dietary modification of saturated fat intake?					
	14. Other					

Weight control and/or loss

Negotiated goals and priorities	P and SO* description	Dates		Dates		Negotiated nursing responsibility, motivational strategies, teaching interventions† (type, date, evaluation and signature)
		Negotiated patient responsibility	Today's results	Negotiated patient responsibility	Today's results	
	1. Describes risks of being overweight or obese with high blood pressure					
	2. Explains how the additional weight places added strain on the heart and vascular system					
	3. Attempts to list reasons for poor eating habits (as applicable)					
	4. States basic four food groups: breads and cereals, milk, meat, fruits and vegetables					
	5. How many servings does he have from each group daily?					
	6. Explains his meal planning and scheduling					
	7. Describes how to utilize low-calorie foods					
	8. Lists ways to manage restaurant eating					
	9. Incorporates low-fat and low-salt diet plans					

*P = Patient; SO = significant others.

†Teaching interventions: 1 = individual counseling; 2 = written materials; 3 = audiovisual presentations; 4 = group sessions.

Continued.

Weight control and/or loss—cont'd

Negotiated goals and priorities	P and SO* description	Dates				Negotiated nursing responsibility, motivational strategies, teaching interventions† (type, date, evaluation and signature)
		Negotiated patient responsibility	Today's results	Negotiated patient responsibility	Today's results	
	10. Indicates family or partner support or nonsupport					
	11. What is today's weight?					
	12. How is he developing new eating habits? Control?					
	13. What are the patient's needs, priorities, desires, and perceptions relative to his weight control or loss?					
	14. Other					

Smoking modification

| Negotiated goals and priorities | P and SO* description | Dates | | Dates | | Negotiated nursing responsibility, motivational strategies, teaching interventions† (type, date, evaluation and signature) |
		Negotiated patient responsibility	Today's results	Negotiated patient responsibility	Today's results	
	1. Lists the effects of smoking on the following: a. Heart b. Lungs c. Brain					
	2. Describes risk of smoking with high blood pressure					
	3. Attempts to list reasons for his smoking practices					
	4. Explains three methods to decrease smoking					
	5. Defines two ways to prevent weight gain while smoking less					
	6. How many packs of cigarettes being smoked daily?					
	7. What are the patient's perceptions, needs, priorities, and desires relative to his smoking practices?					
	8. Other					

*P = Patient; SO = significant others.

†Teaching interventions: 1 = individual counseling; 2 = written materials; 3 = audiovisual presentations; 4 = group sessions.

Alcohol consumption

Negotiated goals and priorities	P and SO* description	Dates			Dates			Negotiated nursing responsibility, motivational strategies, teaching interventions† (type, date, evaluation, and signature)
		Negotiated patient responsibility	Today's results		Negotiated patient responsibility	Today's results		
	1. Lists the effects of alcohol on the following: a. Heart b. High blood pressure c. General health							
	2. Describes risks of drinking alcohol with high blood pressure							
	3. Attempts to explain reasons for patterns of alcohol intake							
	4. Defines three methods to decrease alcohol intake							
	5. What and how many drinks does the patient have a day?							
	6. What are the patient's perceptions, needs, priorities, and desires relative to his alcohol consumption practices?							
	7. Other							

*P = Patient; SO = significant others

†Teaching interventions: 1 = individual counseling; 2 = written materials; 3 = audiovisual presentations; 4 = group sessions.

Hypertension learning resources

HOW TO USE HYPERTENSION CONTROL LEARNING RESOURCES

A comprehensive list of resources for learning about hypertension control is provided. This appendix is divided into sections on the resources for the general public, the patient, and the professional. Usage of the resources depends on cost, time, staff, and facility constraints. In Chapter 6, a description of the counseling process and resource usage is provided. We strongly believe that use of hypertension education resources enhances the patient and family's understanding. However, we do not substitute slides and pamphlets in lieu of individualized counseling by the physician or nurse. We employ them to augment and reinforce the individual and group counseling sessions. Varying the types of materials in a patient education program is necessary to meet individual needs, to progress, and to revise outdated information. Therefore it is necessary to perform ongoing or periodic evaluation. Since cost can be prohibitive at times, we often devise our own pamphlets, charts, and other materials. This can be effective and inexpensive.

During the blood pressure screening and initial evaluation process, we distribute the pamphlets, "High Blood Pressure: What It Is, What It Can Do, What You Can Do About It" (Smith, Kline & French), "Understanding High Blood Pressure" (Searle), "Watch Your Blood Pressure" (Theodore Irwin), and "Stop High Blood Pressure" (Milwaukee County Downtown Hypertension Clinic). Additional materials are distributed as necessary. Initially these comprehensive explanations provide the patient with an overview of hypertension and its control. Furthermore, we show the slide series, "Getting Down On High Blood Pressure: A Patient Education Program" (Milner-Fenwick) at several clinic visits until the patient is well oriented and familiar with hypertension and its treatment. At that point, other materials are used, depending on patient motivation, intelligence, compliance, questions, and need for risk factor modification. Recently a new catalogue has been published that is an excellent source of evaluated publications relevant to hypertension. This is "Educational Materials for Hypertensive Patients: A Catalog of Evaluated Publications" (DHEW Pub. No. [NIH] 77-1244). Other catalogues and sources are available through the National High Blood Pressure Education Program.

The materials have been categorized for use with the general public (undetected populations), treated hypertensives, and professional groups. The sources of media and materials are listed in the last section. Each entry is described according to title, source, and content. Aspects such as technical accuracy, individual audience, treatment and compliance stage usage, and strengths and weaknesses are not included. Reading levels can be assessed by employing the SMOG Readability Formula* or other appropriate tools.

---

*McLaughlin, H.: Smog grading—a new readability formula, J. Read., p. 639, May 1969; and Powers, R. D., et al.: A recalculation of four readability formulas, J. Educ. Psychol. **49**:99, April 1958.

RESOURCES FOR THE GENERAL PUBLIC
Written materials

1. Title: *Don't take chances with high blood pressure*
   Source: High Blood Pressure Information Center
   Content: For black population expressly. Message describes high blood pressure as a silent killer because it is often asymptomatic. *"Knowing* your blood pressure could save your life" could be misleading if nothing is done about it; however, the leaflet encourages detection and treatment.
2. Title: *Get your blood pressure taken before your number's up*
   Source: Department of Health, Education, and Welfare
   Order No. and fee: (HSM) 73-28, none
   Content: General audience. The nature of high blood pressure and who might have it.
   Title: *Tomese la presion antes que le llegue su numero* (Spanish version, same as above)
3. Title: *Health enemy No. 1: High blood pressure/the Merck review*
   Source: Merck, Sharp & Dohme
   Content: Informative comprehensive discussion about the prevalence of high blood pressure as a health problem, its dangers, and description of drugs used to treat it. Message to have regular checkups and spread the word about hypertension.
4. Title: *High blood pressure*
   Source: Citizens for the Treatment of High Blood Pressure
   Content: Brief summary of high blood pressure.
5. Title: *High blood pressure: a positive approach*
   Source: Boehringer Ingelheim Ltd.
   Content: Brief summary of high blood pressure.
6. Title: *HBP is a silent killer*
   Source: Georgia Heart Association
   Content: Flier relates message to get blood pressure checked.
7. Title: *High blood pressure: what it is . . . what it can do . . . what you can do about it*
   Source: Smith, Kline & French Laboratories
   Content: Hypertension, the importance of evaluation and therapy. Well-illustrated and explained discussion of high blood pressure.
   Title: *Presion sanguinea alta: lo que es . . . lo que puede causar . . . lo que usted puede hacer con respecto a la misma* (Spanish version, same as above)
8. Title: *How can high blood pressure hurt you?*
   Source: American Heart Association
   Content: Deals with dangers of undetected high blood pressure, what it is, and need for checkups and following doctor's advice once diagnosed as a hypertensive.
9. Title: *Hypertension—a most misunderstood disease (and word)*
   Source: Merck, Sharp & Dohme
   Content: Briefly defines hypertension, its seriousness, detection, and treatment in simple terminology.
10. Title: *If you love somebody who has high blood pressure—make him take his medicine* (National High Blood Pressure Education Program)
    Source: High Blood Pressure Information Center
    Content: Poster expressly for females addresses itself to compliance in the control of

hypertension with drug therapy by giving some reasons why people stop taking medication. Lists dangers of uncontrolled hypertension. Straightforward, clear.

11. Title: *If you must smoke . . .*
    Source: The Division of Health, Wisconsin Department of Health and Social Services
    Content: Useful suggestions for curtailing and eliminating smoking practices.

12. Title: *"Jimmy the Greek" poster* (16 inches × 21 inches heavy stock)
    Source: Department of Health, Education, and Welfare
    Content: Black and white poster with pocket for information requests. Poster states, "You may not have high blood pressure but I, Jimmy the Greek, say the odds are 10 to 1 you do."

13. Title: *Join the campaign to conquer high blood pressure* (Lawrence Galton)
    Source: Reprint Editor, Reader's Digest
    Content: Brief overview of hypertension control.

14. Title: *Perform a death-defying act*
    Source: American Heart Association
    Content: Straightforward message that encourages public to have blood pressure checked or rechecked.

15. Title: *Understanding high blood pressure*
    Source: Searle & Co.
    Content: Excellent pamphlet with explanatory and simplistic diagrams.
    Title: *Comprendiendo sue presion alta* (Spanish version, same as above)

16. Title: *Volunteer to fight high blood pressure*
    Source: Department of Health, Education, and Welfare
    Content: Outlines essential dangers and controllable nature of high blood pressure. Describes need for volunteers in community programs.

17. Title: *Watch your blood pressure* (Theodore Irwin)
    Source: High Blood Pressure Information Center
    Order No. and fee: Public Affairs Pamphlet No. 483, free, over 50: written distribution plan required
    Content: 28-page booklet provides comprehensive general information about hypertension, including definition, incidence, risk factors, diagnoses, treatment, current research, and preventive action.

18. Title: *Your Blood Pressure*
    Source: American Medical Association
    Content: Describes what blood pressure is, why high blood pressure is not healthy, and how one can tell whether he has it and what can be done.

Audiovisual materials

1. Title: *The brain and hypertension*
   Source: CIBA Pharmaceutical Co.
   Content: (20 min., 16 mm., color, sound)
   The multiple problems and dangers of hypertension as a disease state, with specific reference to the damage incurred by the brain.

2. Title: *The ceaseless heart* (University of Southern California)
   Source: Video Communications, Inc.
   Content: (30 min., videocassette, color, sound)

Presents a discussion of coronary heart disease, high blood pressure, treatment, and prevention as a component of a comprehensive hypertension education program.

3. Title: *Common heart diseases and their causes* (McGraw-Hill)
   Source: American Heart Association
   Content: (17 min., 16 mm., b & w, sound, 1956)
   Animated diagrams clearly explain the circulatory system, how it works, and how it is affected by rheumatic fever, high blood pressure, and arteriosclerosis. Stresses that people with heart disease can lead normal, active lives.

4. Title: *Gameplan life* (Abbott Laboratories)
   Source: Abbott Film Service, Scientificom Distribution Center
   Content: (15 min., 16 mm., color, sound)
   Donald O'Connor in an appealing backstage setting presents the subject of heart attack with reference to his own personal experience. John Hiller, star relief pitcher of the Detroit Tigers and 1974 winner of the Hutchenson Award, joins O'Connor to tell of the pitfalls leading to their heart problems.

5. Title: *The heart and hypertension, 1973*
   Source: CIBA Pharmaceutical Company
   Content: (20 min., 16 mm., color, sound)
   The multiple problems and dangers of hypertension as a disease state, with specific reference to the damage incurred by the heart.

6. Title: *Heart disease—its major causes* (American Heart Association)
   Source: Connecticut State Department of Health
   Content: (11 min., 16 mm., b & w, sound)
   High blood pressure, hardening of the arteries, and rheumatic fever are briefly described. Recent advances in surgical techniques and in the treatment of health disease are shown.

7. Title: *High blood pressure*
   Source: American Heart Association
   Content: (7 min., 16 mm., color, sound)
   Live photographs, diagrams, and animated drawings explain briefly the facts about high blood pressure. Narrator makes it clear that only a physician can tell if high blood pressure is a serious condition and what treatment, if any, is required.

8. Title: *Hypertension*
   Source: Medifact, Inc.
   Content: (8 min. Audiscan and LaBelle cartridges, color, sound)
   Discussion of the nature of hypertension with an explanation of blood pressure. Explains why control of hypertension is of extreme critical importance.

9. Title: *Hypertension and you*
   Source: Lee Creative Communications, Inc.
   Content: (15-16 min., 16 mm., color, sound, 1975)
   Deals with hypertension and the many Americans who are affected by this disease. The disease, its complications, and the way to control it are described. Narrated by Frank Finnerty, Jr., Professor of Medicine, Georgetown University, Washington, D.C.

10. Title: *The pressure is on*

Source: Lee Creative Communications
Content: (9 min., 16 mm., color, sound, 1974)
   Particularly for black audiences, describes what high blood pressure is, how the disease is detected, and its implications. Through animation, the reaction of the body to heart attack, stroke, and kidney failure is illustrated. Narrated by Hugh Morgan of the National Black Network.

11. Title: *Quick, what is your blood pressure?* (Teletronics International, Inc.)
    Source: American Heart Association
    Content: (20 min., 16 mm., color, sound)
       Covers 2-day high blood pressure mass screening during April 1973 in New Orleans. The community effort, dubbed CHEC, for Community Hypertension Evaluation Clinic was sponsored by the Louisiana Heart Association and CIBA Pharmaceutical Co. Stanley B. Garbus, M.D., Specialist in High Blood Pressure Research, Louisiana State University School of Medicine, and James L. Reynolds, M.D., Past President, Louisiana Heart Association, explain the threat of high blood pressure as a major health problem, dangers of complications, and community organization of screening.

12. Title: *Rapid transit for the blood line* (University of Southern California)
    Source: Video Communications, Inc.
    Content: (30 min., videocassette, color, sound)
       Demonstrates blood pressure machine, how the heart pumps blood, and function of red and white blood cells.

13. Title: *Savannah, Georgia: a model community program for hypertension detection and management* (Synthesis Communications, Inc.)
    Source: Mallinckrodt Pharmaceutical Products Division
    Content: (30 min. audio cassette)
       Description of model hypertension program in Savannah, Georgia; how to set up a community detection program.

14. Title: *What goes up?*
    Source: American Heart Association
    Content: (11½ min., 16 mm., color, sound, Spanish/English)
       Observation of 2 men with high blood pressure at an amusement park with their families. One has no symptoms, has high blood pressure, and does not know it because he has not seen a physician in years. The other man has high blood pressure, knows it, and has it under control.

15. Title: *Why risk a heart attack?* (Time-Life)
    Source: Video Communications Associates, Inc.
    Content: (15 min., ½″ and ¾″ cassettes, color, sound)
       Brief, clear presentation to reduce the risk of heart attack; that there are some factors that cannot be controlled and others that can (e.g., tension, diet). Discusses this in industrial context.

16. Title: *Without warning: a story about high blood pressure* (CIBA Pharmaceutical)
    Source: Modern Talking Picture Service, Inc.
    Content: (30 min., 16 mm., color, sound, 1974)
       In personal and dramatic terms, film tells what high blood pressure is and how it can be detected and effectively treated. Story deals with a typical American, his

wife and two children, who works hard. He is one of more than 30 million Americans who have high blood pressure and do not know it. Purpose of the film is to urge all people to get regular blood pressure checks and if found to have hypertension, to get it treated. It also urges those on treatment to stay on treatment for a longer, healthier life.

PATIENT EDUCATION RESOURCES
Written materials

1. Title: *Can we eat well for less?*
   Source: National Dairy Council
   Content: Budget and preparation tips.
2. Title: *Choose your calories by the company they keep*
   Source: National Dairy Council
   Content: Description of basic four food groups and their calories.
3. Title: *Did you take your blood pressure pills today?*
   Source: CIBA Information Services
   Content: Stresses the importance of medication in controlling high blood pressure and the need to continue. Suggests making medication taking a habit and urges keeping medical appointments.
4. Title: *Diet, cholesterol and your heart—there is a connection*
   Source: Lever Brothers Co.
   Content: Explains the relationship between cholesterol and the heart. Discusses low-cholesterol diet and recipes.
5. Title: *Diet of approximately 1,200 calories per day*
   Source: Sandoz Pharmaceuticals
   Content: Daily diet list of 1200 calorie food intake.
6. Title: *Dietary control of cholesterol*
   Source: Fleischmann's Margarines
   Content: Low-saturated fat diet: how to plan, what it is, and who it is for.
7. Title: *Flavor-bright recipes for low-sodium diets*
   Source: General Foods Kitchens
   Content: Hints on the use of Minute Rice and Tapioca in low-sodium diets.
8. Title: *Foods for the low sodium, salt free diet*
   Source: Chicago Dietetic Supply, Inc.
   Content: Brief discussion on foods that are low sodium or salt free. Comprehensive charts giving the sodium content of various foods.
9. Title: *High blood pressure*
   Source: Merck, Sharp & Dohme
   Content: 16-page booklet describes the nature and consequences of high blood pressure, systolic and diastolic pressure, general information on treatment, and the patient's role. Contains pages for notes by the patient on appointment dates, blood pressure readings, and questions for the physician.
10. Title: *High blood pressure and you* (pamphlet and audio cassettes)
    Source: Milwaukee County Medical Complex, DMHS Hypertension Clinic
    Content: Pamphlet written in question-and-answer format fully describing hypertension and treatment. Accompanied by audio cassette series reinforcing pamphlet material.

11. Title: *How doctors diagnose heart disease*
    Source: Superintendent of Documents U.S. Government Printing Office
    Content: Message is as title states: defines the word "diagnosis" and explains methods used in diagnosing heart disease, including blood pressure measurement.

12. Title: *How to stop smoking* (Donald T. Frederickson)
    Source: Alabama Heart Association
    Content: Specific advice on stopping smoking in the form of a 5-week plan. Includes score card and questionnaire on reasons for smoking.

13. Title: *How you can help your doctor treat your high blood pressure* (Marvin Moser, M.D.)
    Source: American Heart Association
    Content: A narrative educational piece for the hypertensive patient. Emphasis on allaying fears and improving compliance.

14. Title: *Hypertension*
    Source: Robert J. Brady Co.
    Content: 24-page, 10 × 13 inch flip chart explaining what blood pressure is, what causes it to be high, and what a hypertensive can do to lower his blood pressure. Take-home materials available.

15. Title: *Hypertension—high blood pressure* (National Heart Institute)
    Source: Superintendent of Documents, U.S. Government Printing Office
    Content: The National Institutes of Health explaining their interest in hypertension and their role in supporting research and training. Facts on hypertension, its causes, diagnosis, dietary and drug treatment, effects of treatment, and patient compliance. Related publication list included.

16. Title: *If you have high blood pressure, don't take chances*
    Source: Department of Health, Education, and Welfare
    Content: Urges regular blood pressure checks and compliance with hypertension control program. Consequences of untreated high blood pressure.

17. Title: *Let's talk about hypertension*
    Source: Bristol Laboratories
    Content: Pamphlet geared toward answering questions of recently diagnosed hypertensives. Prognosis, compliance, and medication and what one can anticipate in terms of life-style are discussed.

18. Title: *Living with high blood pressure* (Article reprint, U.S. News and World Report, October 1974, 4 pages)
    Source: U.S. News and World Report
    Content: Interview with Frank A. Finnerty, Jr., M.D. Discussion of high blood pressure, its complications, factors related to developing the disease, who is most likely to have the disease, methods of treatment, and the need for patient-physician cooperation.

19. Title: *Low cholesterol, fat-controlled recipes*
    Source: Washington Heart Association
    Content: Suggestions for purchasing food, cooking, and dining out. Variety of recipes. Calorie count included.

20. Title: *Low sodium diets*
    Source: General Foods Kitchens
    Content: Discussion of low-salt diet, need, and recipes.

21. Title: *Low sodium diets can be delicious*
    Source: Fleischmann's Margarines
    Content: Booklet explaining low sodium diets includes foods grouped by sodium content levels, menu plans for 1000 mg. sodium diet, and suggested recipes.
22. Title: *Notice! for women only—what are you going to do next year—buy a bigger girdle?*
    Source: The Dairy Council of Wisconsin
    Content: Wall poster.
23. Title: *Obesity* (George Christakis, M.D., and Robert K. Plumb)
    Source: The Nutrition Foundation
    Content: Discourse on cultural factors that impinge on obesity; what obesity is, how individuals develop the condition, formula for weight reduction, the do's and don'ts, and relationship of obesity to good health.
24. Title: *Planning low-sodium restricted meals*
    Source: Robert J. Brady
    Content: Guidelines for planning, preparation, and buying low-sodium foods.
25. Title: *Recipes for fat controlled, low cholesterol meals*
    Source: American Heart Association
    Content: Booklet defines types of fats, cooking tips, and recipes.
26. Title: *Save food $$ and help your heart*
    Source: American Heart Association
    Content: Food budgeting and preparation tips.
27. Title: *Sensible eating can be delicious*
    Source: Standard Brands, Inc.
    Content: General information on basic nutritional counseling.
28. Title: *The silent process—essential hypertension under control*
    Source: Media Medica
    Content: 59-page hardcover textbook. Highly informative for the diagnosed hypertensive or discussion groups. Deals with hypertension and sexuality, complications during pregnancy, and effect on the brain, heart, kidney, and possible changes in medication. For patient understanding and compliance.
29. Title: *Sodium restricted diet: 1000 milligrams*
    Source: American Heart Association
    Content: Discussion of low-salt diet and recipes.
30. Title: *Stop high blood pressure*
    Source: Milwaukee County Medical Complex, DMHS Hypertension Clinic
    Content: Orientation pamphlet designed to facilitate entry of screened hypertensives into treatment.
31. Title: *Straight talk about high blood pressure*
    Source: Merck, Sharp & Dohme
    Content: Stresses hypertensives' role in compliance. Good explanation of physiologic aspects.
32. Title: *The way to a man's heart*
    Source: American Heart Association
    Content: Cholesterol intake and relationship to heart attacks.
33. Title: *Your blood pressure*
    Source: American Medical Association

Content: General patient pamphlet. Discusses blood pressure and hypertension briefly.

34. Title: *Your blood pressure medication, potassium, and diet* (Marvin Moser, M.D., Medical World News, reprint)

    Source: National High Blood Pressure Education Program

    Content: Narrative. Description of hypertension and its treatment.

35. Title: *Your calorie catalog accenting Protein*

    Source: National Dairy Council

    Content: Description of food groups and caloric and protein content.

Audiovisual materials

1. Title: *Childhood hypertension* (Ellin Lieberman, M.D., and Robin Grant, M.P.H.)

   Source: Children's Hospital of Los Angeles

   Content: (8½ min., synchronized slide [73']–tape cassette program, color, sound, 1974, Spanish or English)

   For hypertensive children and their parents.

2. Title: *Choosing life* (Smith, Kline & French Laboratories)

   Source: Walter J. Klein Co., Ltd.

   Content: (15 min., 16 mm., color, sound film)

   A neighborhood pharmacist describes high blood pressure, problems, need for control, that it can be controlled, and consequences if it is not.

3. Title: *Getting down on high blood pressure: a patient education program*

   Source: Milner-Fenwick, Inc.

   Content: (10-15 min. per lesson, 35 mm. filmstrips with automatic cassettes, color, sound, Lesson I-IV)

   Understanding high blood pressure, diet, taking blood pressure medicine, and the "silent killer."

4. Title: *The hard way*

   Source: National High Blood Pressure Information Center

   Content: (30 min., 16 mm., color, sound)

   Bill Cosby narrates. Film follows young black male during screening and treatment for high blood pressure. Emphasizes hypertension, complications, need for compliance, and seriousness for blacks.

5. Title: *High blood pressure*

   Source: Lawren Productions, Inc.

   Content: (50 min., 16 mm. [kinescope], black and white)

   Diagnosis and treatment of high blood pressure and research into causes are illustrated. Emotion, arteriosclerosis, and kidney disorders discussed. Orientation for LPNs and paramedical personnel.

6. Title: *High blood pressure* (Professional Research, Inc.)

   Source: Professional Research, Inc. (PRI) and Video Communications Assoc., Inc.

   Content: (12 min., 16 mm., of Super 8 films, color, sound)

   Describes nature of essential hypertension, that it cannot be cured but it can be controlled, dangers of untreated hypertension, and importance of patient compliance.

7. Title: *How dangerous is high blood pressure?*

   Source: Lawren Productions, Inc.

Content: (11 min., 16 mm., b & w, sound, 1962)
Activity, emotions, food, body weight, and disease may affect blood pressure. Emphasizes medical and dietary management.

8. Title: *Hypertension*
Source: Auburn University
Content: (2 × 2 slide/audio cassette series, 20 min. per lesson, 1974)
Lesson 1: Hypertension—what about it?
Lesson 2: Medication for persons with hypertension
Lesson 3: Eating habits for the control of hypertension
Lesson 4: Exercise
Lesson 5: How to live with your hypertension
Slides in cartoon form; dialogue between "teacher" and "he" and "she."

9. Title: *Hypertension: a delicate balance* (Walter Reed Army Medical Center)
Source: Loan—High Blood Pressure Information Center
Purchase–National Audiovisual Center (GSA)
Content: (10 min., 16 mm., color, sound, 1974)
Patient education film stressing compliance with hypertension drug regimen.

10. Title: *Hypertension and coronary heart disease*
Source: Medfact, Inc.
Content: (12 min., 16 mm., color, sound film or cartridges, color, sound)
A detailed description of hypertension as it relates to coronary disease. Intended in use in patients who are starting a rehabilitation program.

11. Title: *Silent countdown*
Source: Merck, Sharp & Dohme
Content: (16 mm., 30 min., color film)
Features actor Ben Gazzara following the lives of 5 treated hypertensives.

PROFESSIONAL LEARNING RESOURCES
Written materials

1. Title: *The 120/80 notebook for consumer education on high blood pressure*
Source: National High Blood Pressure Education Program
Content: Describes materials, concepts, and organization involved in community control of high blood pressure.

2. Title: *Catalog of audio-visual aids in hypertension*
Source: High Blood Pressure Information Center
Content: Lists audiovisual materials available from a variety of sources.

3. Title: *Children can have high blood pressure too* (D. Greenfield, M.D.)
Source: American Journal of Nursing
Content: Discussion of blood pressure measurement and hypertension in children.

4. Title: *Clinical hypertension* (Norman Kaplan, M.D.)
Source: Medcom, Inc.
Content: Excellent textbook focusing on significant advances in hypertension control

5. Title: *The dentists' role in high blood pressure detection*
Source: Merck, Sharpe & Dohme
Content: Describes the "how" and "why" of starting local high blood pressure detection programs involving dental professionals.

6. Title: *Detecting high blood pressure in an industrial population* (Wallace, Davidson)
   Source: Merck, Sharpe & Dohme
   Content: Describes techniques for industrial-based high blood pressure detection programs.
7. Title: *Directory of national high blood pressure month steering group facilities, May '76.*
   Source: National High Blood Pressure Education Program
   Content: Lists organizations and individuals involved in some manner with the control of high blood pressure.
8. Title: *Education of physicians in high blood pressure*
   Source: National High Blood Pressure Education Program
   Content: Physician's guide on the training and evaluation of physician management of high blood pressure.
9. Title: *Guidelines for HBP control programs in labor organizations*
   Source: Merck, Sharpe & Dohme
   Content: A collection of information, procedures and forms directed at labor organizations to develop high blood pressure control programs.
10. Title: *Guidelines for the evaluation and management of the hypertensive patient*
    Source: National High Blood Pressure Education Program
    Content: Describes basic elements of detection, management, and follow-up.
11. Title: *Guidelines for the use of volunteers for HBP education, detection, and control programs*
    Source: National High Blood Pressure Education Program
    Content: Describes techniques for the utilization of volunteers in the control of high blood pressure.
12. Title: *Handbook of national high blood pressure month, May '76*
    Source: National High Blood Pressure Education Program
    Content: Describes plans, programs, and organizations involved in National High Blood Pressure Education Month, May 1976.
13. Title: *How to avoid pitfalls in measuring BP* (J. Lancour, R.N.)
    Source: American Journal of Nursing
    Content: Discussion regarding proved blood pressure measurement techniques and common errors.
14. Title: *Hypertension*
    Source: Hypertension Publishing Co.
    Content: Discusses issues, research, and publications relevant to HBP.
15. Title: *Hypertension*
    Source: Robert J. Brady Co.
    Content: Patient teaching flip chart, multielement tool.
16. Title: *Hypertension concepts in compliance*
    Source: Abbott Laboratories
    Content: Discusses different aspects of compliance, suggests strategies, and provides clinical simulations.
17. Title: *Hypertension manual: mechanisms, methods, management,* (John Laragh, M.D.)
    Source: Yorke Medical Books

Content: Authoritative review of current medical concepts in hypertension.

18. Title: *Hypertension: mechanisms and management* (Gaddo Onesti, M.D.)
    Source: Grune & Stratton
    Content: The twenty-sixth Hahnemann Symposium discussing treatment of hypertension.

19. Title: *Hypertension: office evaluation*
    Source: American Heart Association
    Content: Discusses high blood pressure and rationale for treatment.

20. Title: *Hypertension: what patients need to know* (M. L. Long, R.N.)
    Source: American Journal of Nursing (**76:**765-770, 1976)
    Content: Hypertension counseling.

21. Title: *Introduction to the nature and management of hypertension* (Edward Freis, M.D.)
    Source: Robert J. Brady Co.
    Content: Describes disease process in detail from anatomy and physiology through treatment programs and practical consideration.

22. Title: *Literature search on hypertension: diagnosis, occurrence and prevention*
    Source: National High Blood Pressure Education Program
    Content: Report on the literature of diagnosis, occurrence, and prevention of high blood pressure. Special emphasis on essential hypertension in the United States.

23. Title: *Literature search on hypertension in the elderly*
    Source: National High Blood Pressure Education Program
    Content: Report on the literature on high blood pressure in the elderly.

24. Title: *Measuring blood pressure*
    Source: Merck, Sharp & Dohme
    Content: Paramedical guide describing technique for measuring blood pressure. Intended for distribution with 16 mm. sound film of the same title.

25. Title: *Program directors' handbook*
    Source: National High Blood Pressure Education Program and Merck, Sharp & Dohme
    Content: Fully details how to develop a community hypertension control program.

26. Title: *The public and high blood pressure summary*
    Source: National High Blood Pressure Education Program
    Content: Summarizes survey results of public awareness and attitudes toward high blood pressure.

27. Title: *Recommendations for human blood pressure determination by sphygmomanometers*
    Source: American Heart Association
    Content: Discusses equipment and techniques to improve accuracy of measurement and reading.

28. Title: *Recurring bibliography of hypertension*
    Source: American Heart Association
    Content: Compiles references from world literature bimonthly.

29. Title: *The R.N.'s goal: under 90 mm. Hg diastolic* (A. Robinson, R.N.; article reprint, R.N. Magazine, May 1974)
    Source: R.N. Magazine
    Content: Discusses challenge of hypertension control to nursing.

30. Title: *Stethoscope convertor*
    Source: Merck, Sharp & Dohme
    Content: Samples of Y-shaped plastic tubing that can be attached to most stethoscopes for training in blood pressure measurement.
31. Title: *The underwriting significance of hypertension for the life insurance company*
    Source: National High Blood Pressure Education Program
    Content: Discusses insurance premiums, hypertension risks, and suggestions for new underwriting policies.

Audiovisual materials

1. Title: *The actions of adrenergic stimulants and antagonists on the cardiovascular system* (Neil C. Moran, M.D.)
   Source: Media Resources Branch
   Content: (20 min., b & w, 16 mm., sound)
   Discusses the actions of experimental drugs on the heart and blood pressure of animals.
2. Title: *Aldosterone: story of a hormone* (G. D. Searle and Co.)
   Source: Media Resources Branch, National Medical Audiovisual Center (Annex)
   Content: (34 min., 16 mm., color, sound, 1969)
   Documents the history of aldosterone through interviews with physicians who pioneered the development of this hormone. Reviews the action of aldosterone in edema and hypertension and shows how knowledge in this subject area is applicable to daily care of patients.
3. Title: *Approach to the patient with elevated blood pressure* (Professional Research, Inc.)
   Source: Video Communications Associates, Inc.
   Content: (30 min., videocassette, color, sound)
   Morton Maxwell, M.D., describes the problems involved with hypertension and how to determine cause and treatment of elevated blood pressure.
4. Title: *Blood pressure readings* (Heart Disease and Stroke Control Program, U.S. Public Health Service)
   Source: Media Resources Branch, National Medical Audiovisual Center (Annex)
   Content: (30 min., 16 mm., color, sound, 1968)
   Shows a manometer with accompanying synchronous Korotkoff sounds for the blood pressure of 14 patients. Tests one's ability to measure blood pressure but does not teach the technique of taking blood pressure.
5. Title: *Blood pressure: theory and process*
   Source: Detroit Education for Nursing Via Television, Wayne State University
   Content: (26 min., 16 mm., [kinescope], b & w, sound)
   Discussion of physiology of blood pressure; the parts, types, and operational principles of equipment; and how to take and record patient's blood pressure.
6. Title: *Cardiovascular physiology, part I* (U.S. Navy)
   Source: Naval Health Services Training and Education Command
   Content: (59 min., ¾" Sony videocassette, b & w, sound, 1971)
   Lecture by Lt. G. Graham, MC, USN, Medical Service, Naval Hospital, NNMC, Bethesda, Md. Introduction to cardiovascular physiology. Discusses functional anatomy and hemodynamics of pressure, volume, and flow.

7. Title: *Cardiovascular physiology, part II* (U.S. Navy)
   Source: Naval Health Services Training and Education Command
   Content: (59 min., helical or ¾" Sony videocassette, b & w, sound, 1971)
   Lecture by Lt. G. Graham, MC, USN, Medical Service, Naval Hospital, NNMC, Bethesda, Md.

8. Title: *Cardiovascular physiology, part III* (U.S. Navy)
   Source: Naval Health Services Training and Education Command
   Content: (50 min., ¾" Sony videocassette, or helical, b & w, sound, 1971)
   Lecture by Lt. G. Graham, MC, USN, Medical Service, Naval Hospital, NNMC, Bethesda, Md.

9. Title: *Childhood hypertension*
   Source: Children's Hospital of Los Angeles
   Content: (8½ min. synchronized slide [73']–tape cassette program, color, sound, 1974, available in Spanish and English)
   Discusses the nature of pediatric hypertension (cause, workup, and therapy) as well as emphasizes how the physician, patient, and family can work together for the best medical management of the patient.

10. Title: *A critical crossroad* (Schering Corp.)
    Source: Association Sterling Films, Inc.
    Content: (28 min., 16 mm., color, sound, 1973)
    Dramatization of a patient in hypertensive crisis treated at Cleveland Clinic for emergency reduction of blood pressure. Clinical aspects of emergency treatment and management of the patient with malignant hypertension are discussed.

11. Title: *Comprehensive management of hypertension*
    Source: Audio-Digest Foundation
    Content: (30-35 min., audio cassettes, 1973)
    Walter Kirkendall, M.D., discusses "The Primary Workup," including major reversible causes and basic laboratory studies, pheochromocytoma, and aldosteronism; and "Therapeutic Approaches," including drug therapy, weight reduction, dietary restrictions, and exercise.

12. Title: *Curable hypertension*
    Source: Audio-Digest Foundation
    Content: (30 min. audio-cassette, 1971)
    Drs. Albert Sokol, Edward G. Biglieri, Harriet P. Dustan, and Edwin J. Wylie discuss aldosterone, renal vascular hypertension, and "What Good are Drugs?" and deal with questions having to do with these subjects. Recorded at the Ninth Scientific Seminar sponsored by Memorial Hospital of Southern California and the Memorial Hospital of Gardena.

13. Title: *Curable hypertension*
    Source: The Network for Continuing Medical Education
    Content: (16 min., videocassette, color, sound)
    With Ralph E. Peterson, M.D., Professor of Medicine and Director, Division of Endocrinology, New York Hospital–Cornell University Medical Center, New York City. Forty million adult Americans have high blood pressure above 150/90 mm. Hg; in half of them hypertension is secondary to another disease process. Surgery is effective in 5% or 1 million of these cases. Dr. Peterson shows how to determine if a hypertensive patient is among the curable million.

14. Title: *Curable hypertension and primary aldosteronism, part I* (Richard H. Edgahl, M.D., and William Hollander, M.D.)
    Source: National Audiovisual Center (GSA)
    Content: (30 min., 16 mm., color, sound)
    Presents the problem of selecting patients from the hypertension group who may have primary aldosteronism. Discusses diagnostic methods.
15. Title: *Curable hypertension and primary aldosteronism, part II* (Paul C. Kahn, M.D., James C. Melby, M.D., and Richard H. Egdahl, M.D.)
    Source: National Audiovisual Center (GSA)
    Content: (30 min., 16 mm., color, sound)
    Discusses therapeutic trial with aldactone and adrenal arteriography as useful additions to workup of hypertension patients.
16. Title: *Current antihypertensive drugs*
    Source: The Network for Continuing Medical Education
    Content: (18 min., videocassette, color, sound)
    G. Victor Rossi, M.D., reviews the basic pharmacologic and toxicologic categories of medicinal agents available for the symptomatic control of hypertension.
17. Title: *Diagnosis and treatment of renal vascular hypertension* (Chester C. Winter)
    Source: American College of Surgeons, Surgical Film Library
    Content: (24 min., 16 mm., color, sound, 1963)
    Complete resume of renal hypertension, including historical factors, important physical examination points, recommended diagnostic screening tests, and further tests once a definite diagnosis has been made. Classification of the lesons causing renal hypertension, treatment of various lesions caused by high blood pressure, and a discussion of prognostic factors are included. No surgical technique is demonstrated.
18. Title: *Diuretics*
    Source: DENT Project (Detroit Education for Nursing Television)
    Content: (22 min., 16 mm., b & w, sound)
    Discusses action of diuretics on kidneys. Identifies nursing responsibilities for patients receiving diuretic drugs.
19. Title: *Drugs used in cardiovascular disease (part I and II)*
    Source: DENT Project
    Content: (Part I, 31 min., 16 mm., kinescope, b & w, sound)
    Identifies five groups of cardiovascular drugs. Discusses actions and uses of cardiac stimulants and cardiac depressants. Identifies and dramatizes nursing responsibilities for patients.
    (Part II, 32 min., 16 mm., kinescope, b & w, sound)
    Discusses actions of vasodilators, vasoconstrictors, and antihypertensives. Identifies and dramatizes nursing responsibilities for patients.
20. Title: *Epidemiology of essential hypertension* (John H. Moyer, M.D.)
    Source: ACCEL (American College of Cardiology Extended Learning)
    Content: (10-15 min. self-assessment exercise)
    Dr. Moyer, one of the earliest to recognize the striking benefit of blood pressure–lowering drugs, in this tape discusses the incidence of hypertension, the characteristics of the hypertensive population with regard to the factors of race, age,

and socioeconomic status. Discussion of the relation of hypertension to atherosclerotic disease and to progressive loss of renal function.

21. Title: *Hazards of hypertension* (Harold M. Adel, M.D., Albert Einstein College of Medicine)
    Source: Albany Medical College
    Content: (30 min., audio cassette with 23 slides)
    Effects of hypertension on the heart, brain, and kidney and danger of treatment.

22. Title: *High blood pressure control: a report from four cities*
    Source: Merck, Sharp & Dohme
    Content: (30 min., 16 mm., color)
    A documentary review of community hypertension detection experiences and techniques in four cities.

23. Title: *How to recognize and treat hypertension*
    Source: Audio-Digest Foundation
    Content: (30 min., audio cassette, 1972)
    Harriet Dustan, M.D., discusses "Evaluation of the Hypertensive Patient" and types of hypertension, George A. Aagaard, M.D., discusses "Medical Treatment of Hypertension," Donald Vidt, M.D., discusses "Hypertensive Emergencies" and treatment, and Howard Morrelli, M.D., discusses "Evaluation of Therapeutic Drugs."

24. Title: *Hyperlipidemias and coronary artery disease: a practical approach* (Frank R. Smith, M.D., and Paul H. Schreibman, M.D.)
    Source: American Heart Association
    Content: (37½ min., 35 mm., audiotape with 23 slides, color)
    Basic steps recommended in the treatment of hypertension and basic methods of management including diet, drug therapy, and indications of types of drugs to be used.

25. Title: *Hypertension—current diagnostic techniques*
    Source: The Network for Continuing Medical Education
    Content: (16 min. videocassette, color, sound)
    New tests developed for differential diagnosis of hypertension. Indications and procedures for these tests are illustrated by Milton Mendlowitz, M.D., Clinical Professor of Medicine and Attending Physician, Mt. Sinai Hospital and Medical Center, N.Y.

26. Title: *Hypertension of adrenal origin—aldosteronism and pheochromocytoma* (Peter H. Forsham, M.D.)
    Source: American Medical Association
    Content: (20 min., 16 mm., color, sound)
    Discussion of two different disorders of the adrenal glands of vital importance, since if diagnosed early, the hypertension caused by them can be cured. In the film, patients with these clinical entities describe their symptomatology. These symptoms are related to the underlying pathology of the disease entity and to the diagnosis. The approach is geared to the working tools available to the practitioner of medicine, particularly history and physical examination. Electrolyte changes and hormonal defects are presented through animation techniques.

27. Title: *Hypertension: the challenge of diagnosis*
    Source: The American Heart Association

Content: (20 min., 16 mm., color, sound)

Demonstrates the approach to diagnosis by posing the two questions that every physician must answer in evaluating a patient with hypertension: What is the cause? What damage has been done? Importance of careful history, physical examination, and selective laboratory procedures to determine whether a primary or a curable form of hypertension is present. Shows the organs most commonly damaged and considers drug treatment of hypertension.

28. Title: *Hypertension update*

Source: Audio-Digest Foundation

Content: (30-35 min., audio cassette, 1974)

This highlight of the American Academy of Family Physicians Twenty-sixth Annual Scientific Assembly, Los Angeles, October 14-17, 1974, features Theodore Cooper, M.D., discussing the "Extent of the Problem"; Ray Gifford, M.D., discussing "Diagnosis and Evaluation"; Louis Tobian, M.D., discussing "Medical Management," including medications; Robert E. Heerens, M.D., covers "Question Topics," including medication side effects and management of hypertensive crisis.

29. Title: *The hypertension workshop* (Medcom)

Source: U.S.V. Pharmaceutical Co.

Content: (25 min., 16 mm., color, sound)

Film: "Dilemmas in Hypertension: Compliance" with Drs. Frank Finnerty, Marvin Moser, Charles Francis, Robert Bilbro, Lois Davis. Physicians in clinic, group, and private practice explain the problem of patient compliance and hypertensive regimens.

Monograph: "A Look at the Treatment of Hypertension" covers the three aspects of treatment: the physician, the patient, and medication, with Drs. Finnerty, Moser, Francis, Bilbro, Davis, and Norman Kaplan.

30. Title: *Hypertensive crisis, part I* (Edward D. Freis, M.D.)

Source: Albany Medical College

Content: (18 min., audio cassette)

Etiology, complications, pathophysiology, clinical evaluation, and laboratory tests.

31. Title: *Hypertensive crisis, part II* (Edward D. Freis, M.D.)

Source: Albany Medical College

Content: (18 min., audio cassette)

Treatment is discussed.

32. Title: *The kidney and hypertension: causes and effects*

Source: South Carolina Regional Medical Program

Content: (58½ min., quadraplex ¾" videotape, b & w, sound, 1971)

Program centers around a discussion dealing with (1) consideration of the kidney as the primary organ involved in high blood pressure, (2) how the kidney affects and is affected by high blood pressure, and (3) importance of control and evaluation of the hypertensive patient.

33. Title: *Long-term effect of hypertensive therapy* (John H. Moyer, M.D.)

Source: ACCEL (American College of Cardiology Extended Learning)

Content: (25 min., ¾" U-Matic cassette, color, sound)

In this tape, Dr. Moyer reviews his accumulation of data over more than twenty years, relating levels of blood pressure to target organ damage, sharing observations of the ganglionic blocking area, and those related to presently available drugs. He reviews the role of small vessel disease of the kidney.

34. Title: *The measurement of blood pressure* (Frances Payne Bolton School of Nursing, Case Western Reserve, under Public Health Grant)
    Source: Media Resources Branch, National Medical Audiovisual Center (Annex)
    Content: (10 min., 16 mm., color, sound, 1971)
    Demonstrates correct procedure for taking blood pressure. Describes mercury sphygmomanometer and its use and the correct reading of systolic and diastolic pressures.

35. Title: *Measuring blood pressure*
    Source: Merck, Sharp & Dohme
    Content: (10 min., 16 mm., color, sound)
    Demonstrates methods of measuring blood pressure and techniques for obtaining more accurate readings.

36. Title: *Mild-to-severe hypertension: tips for treatment*
    Source: The Network for Continuing Medical Education
    Content: (14 min., videotape, color, sound)
    George N. Aagaard, M.D., Professor of Medicine, presents a simple approach to treating patients with hypertension. He outlines the basic nonpharmacologic approach, oral diuretic use, adrenergic inhibitors, smooth muscle dilators, and refractory hypertension.

37. Title: *Modern concepts in hypertension* (David P. Lauler, M.D.)
    Source: Albany Medical College
    Content: (38 min., audio cassette, 67 slides)
    Technique, digitalis status, energy titration, supraventricular tachycardia, atrial flutter and fibrillation, anticoagulation, ventricular tachycardia.

38. Title: *Modern obstetrics: pre-eclampsia, eclampsia* (Wexler Film Productions)
    Source: American Journal of Nursing Company
    Content: (20 min., 16 mm., color, sound, 1972)
    Progression of symptoms from mild preeclampsia to severe eclampsia is clearly presented and the importance of early detection and treatment emphasized. Emergency nature of advanced forms and importance of continuous medical and nursing observation and care stressed. Includes concise delineation of symptoms and treatment with actual patient care situations shown as examples of the three forms of toxemia.

39. Title: *Multiple considerations in managing the hypertensive patient*
    Source: Audio-Digest Foundation
    Content: (25-30 min., audiotape, 1972)
    Ralph Shabetai, M.D., discusses the "Assessment of the Effects and Severity of Hypertension"; Robert G. Luke, M.D., speaks on "Practical Workup for Surgically Remediable Hypertension"; Ray W. Gifford, Jr., M.D., discusses "Drugs for Essential Hypertension." Finally the general therapeutic approach is reviewed.

40. Title: *My hypertensive patient*
    Source: Audio-Digest Foundation
    Content: (45 min., audio cassette)
    Includes speeches presented at June 27, 1973, annual meeting of the American

Medical Association. Discussions are "Classification and Diagnosis of Hypertension," Albert N. Brest, M.D.; "Pharmacologic Treatment," Ray W. Gifford, M.D.; "Hypertensive Encephalopathy," Frank Finnerty, M.D. Drs. Harold T. Dodge, George E. Burch, Edward D. Freis, Brest, Finnerty, and Gifford discuss question topics including how far to go in diagnostic workup, value of taking home blood pressures, diet, and others.

41. Title: *Office management of hypertension* (Marvin Moser, M.D.)
    Source: ACCEL (American College of Cardiology Extended Learning)
    Content: (32 min., ¾″ U-Matic cassette, color, sound)
    Dr. Moser interviews a 37-year-old black male patient who after detection and initial therapy of his hypertension, for various reasons, escaped control and experienced rapid progression of target organ damage.

42. Title: *Patient compliance* (Synthesis Communications, Inc.)
    Source: Mallinckrodt Pharmaceutical Products Division
    Content: (30 min., audio cassette)
    Film is based on the premise that, before a patient can take high blood pressure seriously, the physician must consider it seriously. Patient-physician motivation is dealt with as well as patient-physician communication.

43. Title: *Practical Problems* (Synthesis Communications, Inc.)
    Source: Mallinckrodt Pharmaceutical Products Division
    Content: (30 min., audio cassette)
    Interview of Edward D. Freis, M.D., by Dr. Witten. They discuss problems occurring with high blood pressure, factors to consider before treatment, steps in prescription therapy, side effects and what to do about them, and patient motivation.

44. Title: *Primary hyperaldosteronism, hyporeninemia and hypertension* (James Melby, M.D.)
    Source: Albany Medical College
    Content: (45 min., audio cassette)
    Primary and secondary hyperaldosteronism, plasma aldosterone and renin, use of spironalactone, adrenal venography and blood sampling, and adrenalectomy.

45. Title: *A rational approach to newly discovered hypertension* (revised) (Robert B. Carbeck, M.D.)
    Source: Towsley Center for Continuing Medical Education
    Content: (18 min., audiotape, synchronized with 72 2 × 2″ color slides)
    A rational method of evaluating various cases of newly discovered hypertension on a cost-effective basis is presented with emphasis on the least cost in time and money for both physician and patient.

46. Title: *Reading blood pressure*
    Source: Video Communications Associates, Inc.
    Content: (10 min., ½″ videotape, videocassettes, color, sound)
    Describes and shows how to take blood pressure readings.

47. Title: *Reconstructive surgical procedures for renal arterial stenosis with hypertension* (Paul T. DeCamp, M.D.)
    Source: American College of Surgeons
    Content: (33 min., 16 mm., color, sound, 1961)
    Film contains the surgical techniques involved in four different methods of recon-

structive arterial surgery for renal arterial stenosis associated with hypertension. Included are resection and direct anastomosis, a plenorenal and arterial shunt, an endarterectomy, and an aortorenal plastic bypass graft.

48. Title: *Renal angiography in hypertension: transfemoral artery technique* (Robert G. Weaver, M.D.)

    Source: American College of Surgeons

    Content: (25 min., 16 mm., sound, color, 1961)

    Explains author's method of diagnosing lesions, with particular emphasis on angiography by the transfemoral artery technique.

49. Title: *Renal factors in blood pressure regulation*

    Source: Professional Communications, The Upjohn Co.

    Content: (4¾ min., 16 mm., color, sound, 1965)

    Irvine Page, M.D., codiscoverer of angiotensin, explains the derivation of the name. This is followed by an animated illustration of the renin-angiotensinogen-angiotensin I-angiotensin II-aldosterone chain of events. When occlusive renovascular disease produces the Goldblatt clamp effect, surgery may be required to reduce the resulting blood pressure. The various types, ranging from endarterectomy to bilateral nephrectomy, are outlined.

50. Title: *Renal hypertension/bilateral nephrectomy/kidney transplantation* (W. J. Kolff, I. H. Page, M.D., and H. Goldblatt, M.D.)

    Source: American Heart Association

    Content: (23 min., 16 mm., color, sound, 1965)

    Medical report designed to bring physicians, regardless of specialty, up-to-date on the recent development in the management of renal hypertension, including indications and contraindications, clinical results to date, and future possibilities.

51. Title: *Renal vascular hypertension: an approach to diagnosis and treatment* (Harry E. Sarles, M.D.)

    Source: Media Resources Branch, National Medical Audiovisual Center (Annex)

    Content: (20 min., 16 mm., color, sound)

    Demonstrates the pathogenesis and diagnosis of renal vascular hypertension and the types of lesions possible.

52. Title: *The role of adrenal cortex in hypertension* (Grant Liddle, M.D.)

    Source: Albany Medical College

    Content: (43 minutes, audio cassette)

    Presents relationship of steroids to hypertension and how to diagnose. Suggests a method of treatment.

53. Title: *Selective renal angiography* (Murray C. Baron and Herbert Brendler)

    Source: American College of Surgeons

    Content: (10 min., 16 mm., color, sound, 1965)

    Selective renal angiography is a safe and simple technique offering valuable diagnostic information regarding lesions of the kidney not available by other methods. The method of percutaneous femoral puncture is first illustrated in animated drawings; actual technique of selective renal artery catheterization is then demonstrated in its entirety.

54. Title: *Sodium restricted diets* (Sr. M. Perpetua Reis, M.S., R.D., and Ann Ruggiero, B.S., R.D.)

Source: Albany Medical College

Content: (18 min., audiocassette, 6 slides)

Types of sodium restricted diets; use in pregnancy and geriatrics; need for patient education.

55. Title: *Surgical treatment of renovascular hypertension* (George C. Morris, Jr., M.D., Michael E. DeBakey, M.D., E. Stanley Crawford, M.D., Denton A. Cooley, M.D.)

Source: American College of Surgeons

Content: (25 min., 16 mm., color, sound, 1960)

Documents development of more precise diagnostic methods together with improved techniques in vascular surgery that have stimulated new interest in this treatment of renovascular hypertension. Essential features in the diagnosis, physiology, pathology, and surgical treatment are presented.

56. Title: *Surgical treatment of renovascular hypertension* (Chester C. Winter, M.D.)

Source: American College of Surgeons

Content: (25 min., 16 mm., color, sound, 1962)

The problem of renovascular hypertension is shown, including its diagnosis, laboratory evaluation, and surgical correction. In the first case the renal occlusion is removed and patch graft applied. A second case illustrates surgical correction by Dacron tube grafts.

57. Title: *Treatment of the hypertensive patient* (John H. Moyer, M.D.)

Source: ACCEL (American College of Cardiology Extended Learning)

Content: (46 min., ¾″ U-Matic cassette, color, sound)

Comprehensive review of the pharmacology of currently used blood pressure–lowering drugs, including mechanism of action, untoward effects, and details of proper use.

58. Title: *Treatment of moderate hypertension* (Harriet P. Dustan, M.D.)

Source: Albany Medical College

Content: (17 min., audio cassette)

Value and reasons of treatment; a method of approach.

59. Title: *Vital signs, part 3* (U.S. Navy)

Source: Naval Health Sciences Education and Training Counsel

Content: (11 min., 16 mm., b & w., color, sound)

Explains the principles behind taking blood pressures. Demonstrates procedures followed with patients. Uses sound effects to show the significant changes in pulse tone.

60. Title: *When should hypertension be treated?*

Source: The Network for Continuing Medical Education

Content: (19 min., videotape, color, sound)

Edward Freis, M.D., and Ray W. Gifford, Jr., M.D., review through patient interviews the recent changes in criteria for intervention in hypertension.

ADDITIONAL SOURCES OF MEDIA AND MATERIALS
Government agencies

Connecticut State Department of Health
Public Health Education Section
79 Elm St.
Hartford, Conn. 06115

Department of Health, Education, and
Welfare
National Medical Audiovisual Center
Atlanta, Ga. 30333

Department of Health, Education, and
Welfare
National Medical Audiovisual Center
(Annex)
Station K
Atlanta, Ga. 30324

Division of Health
Wisconsin Department of Health and
Social Services
Box 309
Madison, Wis. 53701

High Blood Pressure Information Center
120/80 National Institutes of Health
Bethesda, Md. 20014

National Audio-Visual Center (GSA)
Sales Branch
Washington, D.C. 20409

Naval Health Sciences Education and
Training Command
Media Resources Librarian
Media Department
National Naval Medical Center
Bethesda, Md. 20014

State Board of Health
Florida State Board of Health
Jacksonville, Fla. 32202

Superintendent of Documents
U.S. Government Printing Office
Washington, D.C. 20402

Veterans Administration
Central Office Film Library

Audio Visuals Service
Washington, D.C. 20420

Nonprofit organizations

Alabama Heart Association
706½ South 29th St.
Birmingham, Ala. 35233

American College of Surgeons
Surgical Film Library
Davis and Geck Distributors
1 Casper Street
Danbury, Conn. 06810

American Heart Association
Film Library
267 West 25th St.
New York, N.Y. 10001

American Hospital Supply
2020 Ridge Ave.
Evanston, Ill. 60201

American Medical Association
535 N. Dearborn St.
Chicago, Ill. 60610

Children's Hospital of Los Angeles
P.O. Box 54700
Los Angeles, Calif. 90054

Citizens for the Treatment of High Blood
Pressure, Inc.
Suite 1630, Chevy Chase Bldg.
5530 Wisconsin Ave.
Chevy Chase, Md. 20015

Dairy Council of Wisconsin
9898 W. Bluemound Rd.
Milwaukee, Wis. 53226

Florida Heart Association
St. Petersburg, Fla. 33733

Georgia Heart Association
2581 Piedmont Rd., N.E.
Atlanta, Ga. 30324

Hypertension Clinic
Milwaukee County Medical Complex
2430 W. Wisconsin Ave.
Milwaukee, Wis. 53233

National Dairy Council
Rosemont, Ill. 60018

Nutrition Foundation
888 17th St., N.W.
Washington, D.C. 20406

Washington Heart Association
2007 Eye St., N.W.
Washington, D.C. 20006

Pharmaceutical firms

Abbott Laboratories
Medical Department
14th St. and Sheridan Rd.
North Chicago, Ill. 60064

Ames Co.
Division of Miles Laboratories, Inc.
Elkhart, Ind. 46514

Baxter Laboratories
Morton Grove, Ill. 60053

Bristol Laboratories
Division of Bristol-Myers Company
Syracuse, N.Y. 13201

CIBA Pharmaceutical Co.
556 Morris Ave.
Summit, N.J. 07901

Claremont Medical Laboratory
370 West Third St.
Claremont, Calif. 91711

Eaton Laboratories
17 Eaton Ave.
Norwich, N.Y. 13815

Eli Lilly & Co.
Audio-Visual Film Library
Box 618
Indianapolis, Ind. 46206

E. R. Squibb & Sons, Inc.
Professional Service Department

745 Fifth Ave.
New York, N.Y. 10022

G. D. Searle & Co.
Reference & Resource Program
1841 Broadway
New York, N.Y. 10023

Geigy Pharmaceuticals
Medical Service Department
Box 430
Yonkers, N.Y. 10702

Lederle Laboratories
Medical Advisory Department
Pear River, N.Y. 10965

*Mallinckrodt Pharmaceutical Products
    Division*
434 North Morgan St.
Decatur, Ill., 62525

William S. Merrell Co.
Department of Professional Relations
Cincinnati, Ohio 45215

Merck, Sharp & Dohme
Professional Services Department
West Point, Pa. 19486

Pfizer Laboratories
Professional Services Department
235 East 42nd St.
New York, N.Y. 10017

Roche Laboratories
Professional Service Department
Nutley, N.J. 07110

*Ross Laboratories—Division of Abbott
    Laboratories*
Columbus, Ohio 43215

Sandoz Pharmaceuticals
Medical Film Department
Rt. 10
Hanover, N.J. 07936

Searle & Co.
San Juan, P.R. 00936

Smith, Kline & French Laboratories
Medical Department

1500 Spring Garden St.
Philadelphia, Pa. 19101

Upjohn Professional Film Library
7000 Portage Road
Kalamazoo, Mich. 49001

Professional Communication
Upjohn Company
7000 Portage Rd.
Kalamazoo, Mich. 49001

U.S.V. Pharmaceutical Company
1 Scarsdale Rd.
Tuckahoe, N.Y. 10707

Winthrop Labs
Medical Film Department
90 Park Ave.
New York, N.Y. 10016

Wyeth Laboratories
Professional Service
Box 8299
Philadelphia, Pa. 19101

Educational facilities

Albany Medical College
47 New Scotland Ave.
Albany, N.Y. 12208

*American College of Cardiology Extended
  Learning (ACCEL)*
9650 Rockville Pike
Bethesda, Md. 20014

Auburn University
Education Television Department
Auburn, Ala. 36830

Center for Mass Communications
Columbia University Press
440 W. 110th St.
New York, N.Y. 10025

Indiana University
Audio Visual Center
Bloomington, Ind. 47401

*The Network for Continuing Medical
  Education*

15 Columbus Circle
New York, N.Y. 10023

New York University College of Medicine
550 First Ave.
New York, N.Y. 10016

*South Carolina Regional Medical
  Program*
Medical University of South Carolina—
  Division of Continuing Education
80 Barre St.
Charleston, S.C. 29401

*Towsley Center for Continuing Medical
  Education*
University of Michigan
Ann Arbor, Mich. 48104

University of Wisconsin at Milwaukee
Robert E. Norris Health Center
2416A E. Hartford Ave.
Milwaukee, Wis. 53211

Publishers and audiovisual producers

Abbott Film Service
Scientificom Distribution Center
708 North Dearborn
Chicago, Ill. 60610

American Journal of Nursing Co.
Educational Sources Division
Film Library
267 West 25th St.
New York, N.Y. 10001

Association Films, Inc.
Source for American Hospital Association
  Films
512 Burlington Ave.
La Grange, Ill. 60525
        or
8615 Directors Row
Dallas, Texas 75247

Association Sterling Films, Inc.
512 Arlington Ave.
La Grange, Ill. 60525

Audio Digest Foundation
1250 S. Glendale Ave.
Glendale, Calif. 91205

Bailey Film Association
11559 Santa Monica Blvd.
Los Angeles, Calif. 90025

Blakiston's Audiovisual Materials
McGraw-Hill Book Co.
330 West 42nd St.
New York, N.Y. 10036

Boehringer Ingelheim, Ltd.
Elmsford, N.Y. 10523

Robert J. Brady Co.
130 Que St., N.E.
Washington, D.C. 20002

Burgess Publishing Co.
Audio Tutorial Systems
426 South Sixth St.
Minneapolis, Minn. 55415

Carousel Films, Inc.
Suite 1503
1501 Broadway
New York, N.Y. 10036

Communications Division
University of Nebraska
College of Medicine
602 South 44th Ave.
Omaha, Neb. 68105

Concept Media
1500 Admas Ave.
Costa Mesa, Calif. 92626

*Detroit Education for Nursing via
    Television (DENT)*
College of Nursing
Wayne State University
Detroit, Mich. 48202
            and
American Journal of Nursing Co.
Educational Services Division
Visual Information Systems Center for
    Videotape

15 Columbus Circle
New York, N.Y. 10023

Filmmakers Library, Inc.
11 Riverside Dr.
New York, N.Y. 10023

Grune & Stratton
111 Fifth Ave.
New York, N.Y. 10003

Health Film Association
15533 S.E. Ninth St.
Bellevue, Wash. 98004

Hypertension Publishing Co.
79 Madison Ave.
New York, N.Y. 10016

International Film Bureau
332 S. Michigan Ave.
Chicago, Ill. 60604

Walter J. Klein Co., Ltd.
3601 Carmel Rd.
Charlotte, N.C. 28211

Lawren Productions, Inc.
P.O. Box 1542
Burlingame, Calif. 94010

Lee Creative Communications, Inc.
P.O. Box 1367
Rochester, N.Y. 14603

J. B. Lippincott Co.
East Washington Square
Philadelphia, Pa. 19105

MedCom, Inc.
Multimedia Medical Education Programs
2 Hammarskjold Plaza
New York, N.Y. 10017

Medfact, Inc.
P.O. Box 458
420 Lake Ave., N.E.
Massillon, Ohio 44646

Medi Visuals, Inc.
342 Madison Ave.

Suite 1812
New York, N.Y. 10017

Media Medica
4 Midland Ave.
Hicksville, N.Y. 11801

Milner-Fenwick, Inc.
3800 Liberty Heights Ave.
Baltimore, Md. 21215

Modern Talking Picture Service, Inc.
2323 New Hyde
New Hyde Park, N.Y. 11040

Prentice Hall
Englewood Cliffs, N.J. 07632

Professional Research, Inc. (PRI)
660 S. BonnieBrae St.
Los Angeles, Calif. 90057

Reprint Editor
Reader's Digest
Pleasantville, N.Y. 10570

R.N. Magazine
Reprint Department
550 Kinderkanack Rd.
Oradell, N.J. 07649

Trainex Corp.
P.O. Box 116
Garden Grove, Calif. 92642

U.S. News and World Report
2300 North St., N.W.
Washington, D.C. 20037

Video Communications, Inc.
Suite 904, Watergate Office Bldg.
2600 Virginia Ave., N.W.
Washington, D.C. 20037

John Wiley & Sons, Inc.
605 Third Ave.
New York, N.Y. 10016

York Medical Books
Dun-Donnelly Publishing Corp.
New York, N.Y. 10003

Industries

Chicago Dietetic Supply, Inc.
P.O. Box 40
La Grange, Ill. 60525

Fleischmann's Margarine
625 Madison Ave.
New York, N.Y. 10022

General Foods Kitchens
250 North St.
White Plains, N.Y. 10605

Lever Brothers Co.
Box 1385
Clinton, Idaho 52734

Standard Brands
625 Madison Ave.
New York, N.Y. 10022

INDEX